DIY Care and Repair of Stylist Shears

A Manual for Every Hair Cutting Scissor Owner

Bonnie Megowan

Copyright © 2019 Bonnie Megowan

All rights reserved.

ISBN: 9781099613388

DEDICATION

Dedicated to my family.

My husband Gene Megowan of 43 years of marriage and 30 years of business has encouraged me to do more, be more and learn more. He is my cheerleader and council throughout all my endeavors. He reminds me of our company mission statement *to glorify Christ and to deal with our business associates as we would want them to deal with us.*

Also dedicated to the rest of my family which includes my daughters, grandchildren and in-laws, especially Mystie who blocked interruptions while I worked on my book and Susannah who took many of the photos.

Beyond my related family, I dedicate this book to my extended business family; the stylists who use our shears and their sharpeners.

Chapter	Contents	Page
	Introduction	1
1	Know Your Cutting Personality	4
2	Understanding Your Shears	7
3	Running with Shears	19
4	Don't Have a Loose Screw	23
5	How to Clean Your Shears	32
6	How to Fight Rust	36
7	How to House Your Shears	40
8	How to Replace Finger Rests	47
9	How to Replace Bumpers	50
10	How to Make Your Shears Fit	55
11	How to Tell if Your Shears are Dull	60
12	How to Find a Sharpener	68
13	Specialty Shears DIY Tips	77
14	Conclusion	87
	About the Author	91

Introduction

This book on *DIT Care and Repair of Stylist Shears* will guide you through the care and simple repairs of typical beauty shears. Following these guidelines, if you own 4 or more pairs of shears, the information in this book will save you possibly thousands of dollars in their career.

Reading this book will show you how to prolong the life of your shears and go longer between sharpening. Too frequent sharpening ages your shears and is the leading reason for shear replacement.

You will not learn how to fire your professional shear sharpener by reading this book. There will be times when your only alternative is to call the shear service expert. You will, however, learn some of the knowledge, skills, tools and supplies the professionals use. You will also learn *Do It Yourself* ways to do what they do. Many of the hacks utilize simple items you probably already have in your salon, purse or pocket.

IN THIS BOOK YOU WILL LEARN THE FOLLOWING:

- What is your Cutting Personality and how that affects the care of your shears
- How to talk intelligently to your sharpener or shear rep using the correct terminology and shears parts that they use
- How to avoid cuts and injuries by using some common sense shear safety
- How to correctly adjust your pivot screw
- How to correctly clean your shears
- How to store your shears between use and for transport
- How to prevent rust on your shears and preserve the shine
- How to replace the finger rest and hacks to use if you don't have one
- How to replace the bumper or spacer between the handle and hacks if you don't have one
- How to make the shears fit your fingers
- What are the 3 types of edges on shears
- How to tell if your shears are dull
- How to bring back the edge
- When to call a shear sharpening expert
- How to select a shear sharpener
- What to do if there is not a sharpener in your area
- DIY care for specialty shears – curved shears, texturizers and thinners, left handed shears

1

KNOW YOUR CUTTING PERSONALITY

Before you begin any *"Do It Yourself"* care and repair of your expensive beauty shears it is best to understand yourself and your approach to what you will learn in this book. As a sharpener, former high school science teacher and an observer of stylists cutting hair, I have noticed that most hair cutters will fall into one of three categories of cutting personalities. I named these after animals. Each of these personalities will have a different approach to shear care and how they use this book.

Eagles

Eagles are beautiful creatures. They are graceful to watch as they soar through the sky. They are precise as they target their prey and slice through the air. Most cosmetology instructors are eagles which means cosmetology students are most often taught to cut like eagles, even if they have developed into another animal as their career progressed.

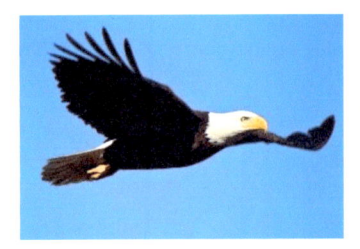

I am assuming most of you reading this are *Eagles.* Eagles are the most particular about their shears and will take the time to learn more about them. The eagles will get the most benefit out of the chapters on caring for their shears and probably do very little in the repair department unless they can't locate a sharpener.

Eagles don't usually own a lot of shears but what they have are good and sometimes they like to use the same shears for years. They will take notice of any changes in the way their shears cut. Eagles will hold their shears with a lighter grip, use a palm to palm cutting position and take clean narrow partings when cutting. They cut slower but with more precision. They can repeat the same hair cut time after time since they are aware of their body position and stance as they execute a cut. Their station is neat, the floor is swept, and their tools are clean.

Eagles will read this book cover to cover, front to back.

Lions

If you are a lion, you go to lots of hair shows and you try anything new. You love to watch videos by of salon educators and take cutting classes.

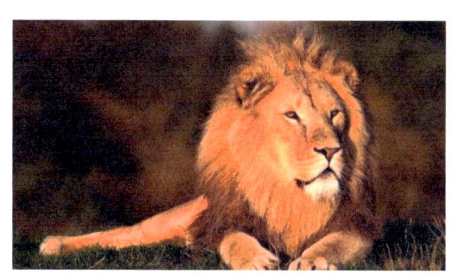

Lions will skip around in this book and read the highlights, chapter titles and dwell on any DIY sections. They will relish the repairs and will try all the repairs on their shears. They have a lot of repairs because they have a lot of shears and don't always care for them properly.

Lions are brave. They will risk a bad shear repair or even a bad haircut in order to try something new. Their station is organized to their eyes but cluttered looking to others. They like innovative tools, fresh ideas and are energized by anything new and shiny.

Lions will be the first to buy this book but never read all of it. They will get the gest by skimming the highpoints.

Gorillas

Gorillas are highly intelligent, playful and innovative. They are strong with strong hands. They follow their heart in planning their day.

You are probably not a gorilla. If you are, you are equipping yourself to teach rather than gathering knowledge about your shears. Very few gorillas will be reading this book unless they know me as the author or they are teaching haircutting and shear care.

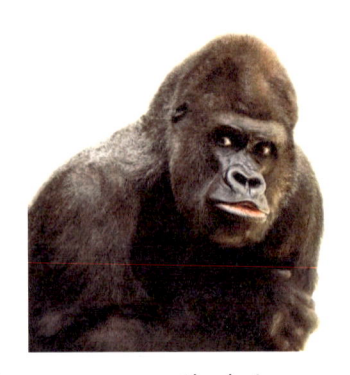

Gorillas are movers and shakers. They don't take the time to care for their shears, much less read a book about it. Over the years they have bought a lot of shears but they don't own a lot because they are lost, stolen or damaged beyond use. Their station is a mess. They don't always sweep up the hair.

If the gorillas utilize this book, they will use it as a reference skipping to the sections on shear repair when their shears stop working. Because they never clean, oil or adjust their shears, their shears need more repairs than most. Combine that with the fact that they cut big chunks of hair, cut fast and hold their shears with a "gorilla" grip; the handles can become mangled, bumpers pop off and the teeth of their texturizers start biting into the other blade.

Gorillas can benefit from the information here but will probably benefit more from a local sharpener who understands the creative side of the gorilla and keeps their shears working without judgment.

2

UNDERSTANDING YOUR SHEARS / SCISSORS

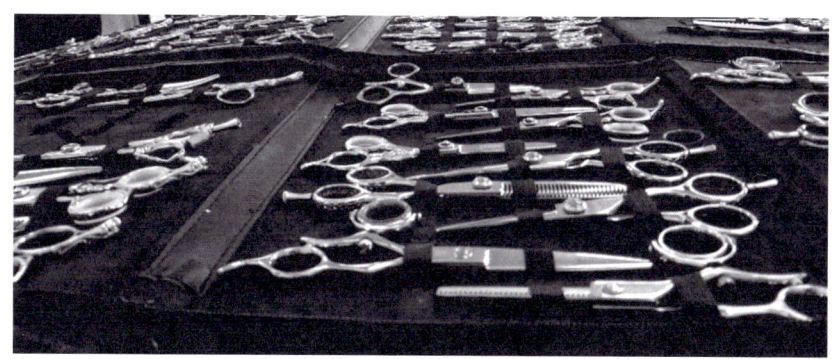

Which is it? Shears or Scissors? Scissors or Shears? If you are in the United States or Canada the typical stylist will call them shears. Other countries generally refer to them as scissors, although Australia and New Zealand are beginning to use the word "shears."

The dictionary will tell you that a shear must be longer than 6 inches and scissors are shorter. When I began sharpening in the 80's both terms were used, but the younger stylists, particularly those with Japanese style shears called them shears. I don't know the exact etymology of the word, but it seems that when the convex shaped blade debuted, this is when the transition was made between the name scissors to shears. When asked what is the difference between scissors and shears, I normally quip, "About $100.00."

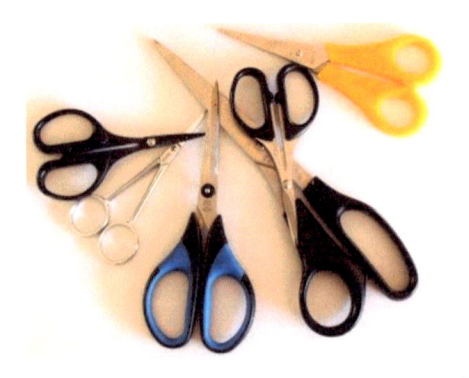

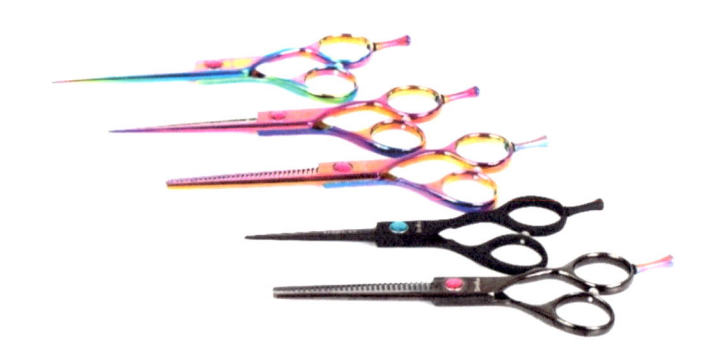

Another question I am asked is why are the words scissors and shears plural. This is because there are two blades that are attached. They are always called a "pair" of shears or a "pair" of scissors. Once again, the grammatical term for these tools is always in the plural, in the common everyday usage by stylists they may refer to their tool as either a shear or a pair of shears and sometimes my scissor or a pair of scissors.

In the early days of my sharpening, I ran an ad in a local paper advertising I would sharpen a pair of shears for X amount of dollars. I received a call to sharpen two pairs of shears. When I gave her the bill, the stylist only wanted to pay half the amount because I had advertised to sharpen a pair of shears, not just one shear. I can't remember now if I gave her a free sharpening that day or not. I do remember giving her a mini-lesson on the correct grammar and terminology for her tools. Once a schoolteacher, always a schoolteacher.

Now that you know what to call your tool you should also know the names for the parts of your shears. There is no way to communicate with your shear rep or sharpener without knowing what to call the *thingy* on the *thing* of your shears. If you have a problem and you are unable to explain what issue you are having it is hard to find the solution to your problem.

Unfortunately, the terminology on shear parts learned in cosmetology school has very little relation to the world of shear sharpeners. Pick up your textbook from cosmetology school and you will find a diagram with the parts of your shears labeled. Pick up the textbook from the stylist in the next chair and you will find a different set of labels. If you go on the internet and look at diagrams the same part may be called a nail hole, pivot hole, neck, vortex and any number of names. Just the finger rest alone can be called the tang, pinky rest, finger hook or *that thing that keeps falling off the end of my shears.*

These are the parts of the shears with terms most commonly used by USA sharpeners and international sharpeners who trained in America. They are not necessarily the correct terms as used by the manufacturer, but they are the terms that will help you communicate most effectively with your sharpener should the occasion arise and will help you with the instructions and explanations of this book. Please refer to them as needed as you move through the chapters.

1. Finger hole
2. Shank – This is an offset style shear where one shank is longer than the other shank.
3. Pivot screw – This pivot screw in this photo is a thumb-nut type pivot screw.
4. Inside the blade – This blade has a *hollow grind* which means it has a concave shape inside the blade.
5. Cutting edge – This particular shear has a convex or Japanese style cutting edge.
6. Rideline – Some sharpeners may call it a hone or hone line. This is the shiny surface along the edge of Japanese type shears that allow the blades to glide over each other.
7. Tip or point
8. Spine or Back of the blade – This is the side of the blade that is not sharp.
9. Outside blade – This is the part of the blade that shows when the shears are closed.
10. Insert ring or sizer – These are plastic rings that pop in the holes to make the shears fit your fingers better.
11. Bumper – This a small piece usually made of plastic that separate the handles so the shear is quieter and less jarring to the hand when you close the shear. I have seen these called spacers, silencers, and stop buffer.
12. Half Moon or Ride – This is the back semicircle behind the pivot screw. This is the area commonly oiled.
13. Logo – The brand of the shear is usually found in this spot. The model number and size can normally be found on the opposite side. This section may be called the "joint" by scissor manufacturers.
14. Finger Rest – This one is a removeable tang, some shears have a *fixed tang*.

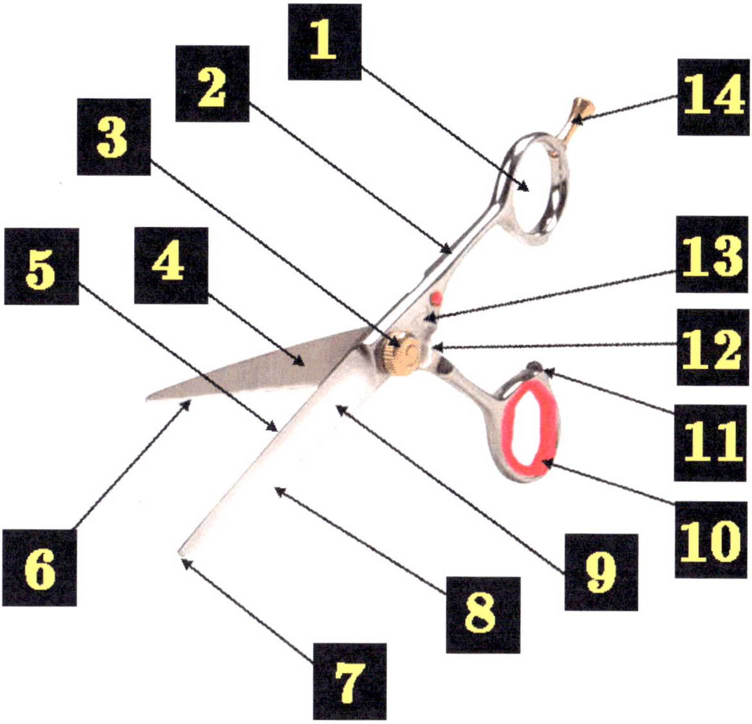
1
2
3
4
5
6
7
8
9
10
11
12
13
14

Shear Edges

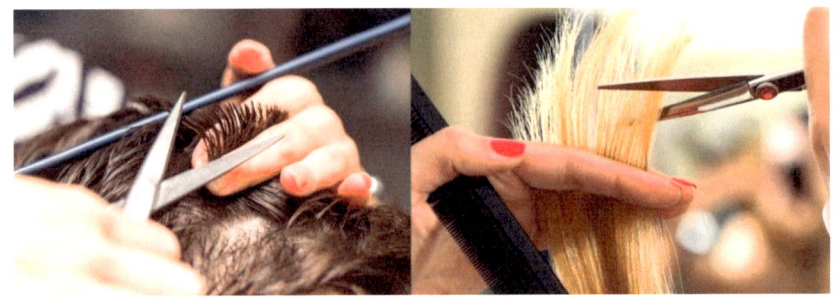

Left figure: German barber style beveled edge. Right figure: Asian beauty style convex edge.

There are two basic styles of shear edges. Most USA stylists shears are an Asian or Japanese style. They have a soft, quiet cut. They are usually sharper, but need sharpening more often. Others are European or German style. These have a stiffer, crisper feel. They will go for a longer time without sharpening. The two styles are determined by the edge put on the shears. The German style shears are what sharpeners in the USA call a beveled edge.

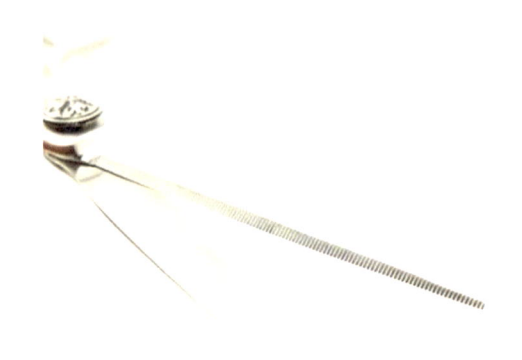

Bevel edge shear

The beveled edge blade is flat. Sometimes one or both edges will have tiny teeth or ridges called serrations. These keep the hair from pushing even when the blades dull. There will be a whooshing sound when the shears close.

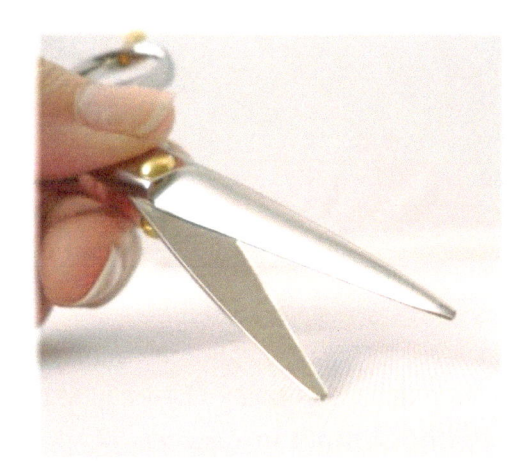

Convex edge shear

An Asian style shear is typically a convex edge. If you were to cut the blade in half the edge would look like a clam shell. The surface of the outside of the blade gently curves to the cutting edge so that there is not a distinct line where the blade slopes to the edge. The inside of the blade will be concave or hollow ground with a shiny line running along the inside of the edge. This is called the rideline. The edges on a convex edge shear are normally sharper and they will give a cleaner cut with less chance of split ends.

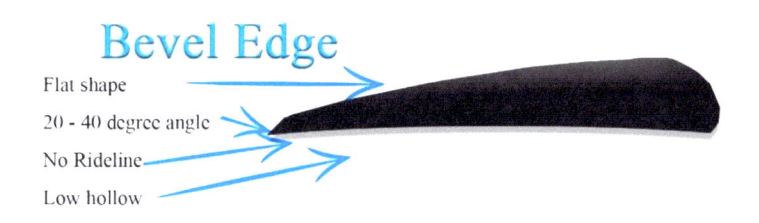

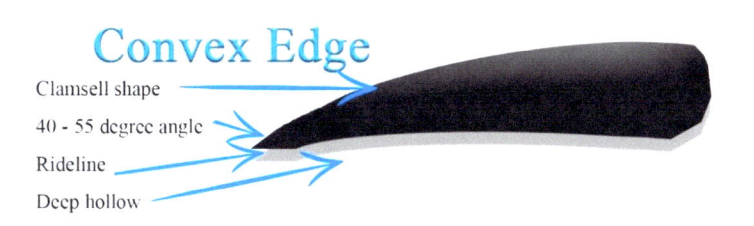

Bevel Edge
- Flat shape
- 20 - 40 degree angle
- No Rideline
- Low hollow

Convex Edge
- Clamsell shape
- 40 - 55 degree angle
- Rideline
- Deep hollow

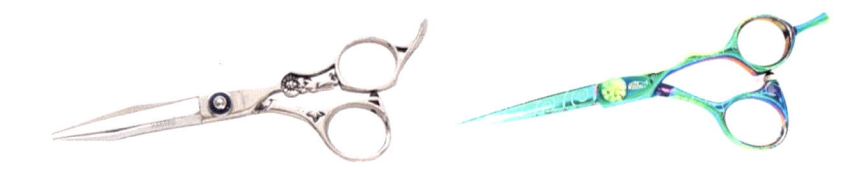

Left: Sword Edge shear. Right: Colored coated shear

There are some hybrid shears as well. Shears with a color have a semi-convex or micro bevel. The cutting edge is sharpened after the color is applied and there is a small beveled area. These may or may not have the hollow grind with a rideline. There are also sword edge shears which have a very sharp and wide bevel. These would have the hollowgrind on the inside of the blade and a rideline as well.

Shear Handles

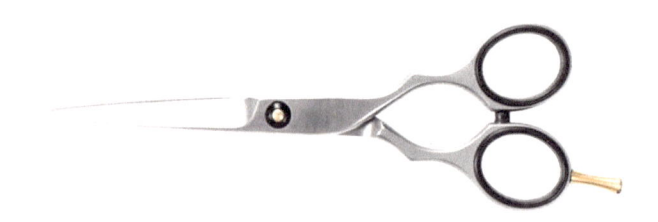

Above: Even handle. Below: Offset handle

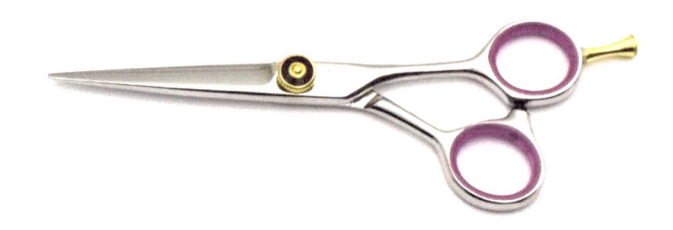

Shears will have different style handles Once again there are two basic styles with one major variation. The even or straight handle shears with shanks the same length are sometimes called traditional handles. These are seen more commonly with barbers and European stylists. The other basic handle is the offset handle which is more common in stylist shears sold in the United States. The shank on one side is longer than the other. Offset handles are more ergonomic for those who cut palm to palm or thumb down. The variation on these two handle styles is the swivel thumbs or twisters. These shears have a thumb hole that rotates or rocks to give a more relaxed cut. The shears with a swivel can be difficult to get used to, but are the most comfortable for the hand with less hand cramps than other shears.

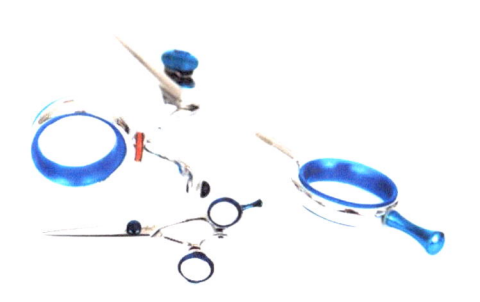

Swivel thumb handle or "Twister" shear

DIY Idea: What can you do if the screw comes out on your swivel thumb shear and you can't put it back?

Push a paper clip or tie wrap through the holes and secure in place until you can get a professional repair done.

If you have the screw and it keeps coming unscrewed, apply some nail polish or nail glue to the threads and screw back into place. Let the glue dry. Use the shear until you can get a professional repair.

Shear Colors and Design

Shears can be very beautiful and ornate. They can also be very classic and austere. Selections are many, with a rainbow of colors and finish. Some have decorative handles and fancy pivot screws. Remember when you are selecting your shears, all these designs are window dressing. Some may even interfere with the quality of the steel and the comfort of the handle. Beauty is important. My husband says that's why he selected me, although I think it was my brains. Real quality is based on the choice of steel and the workmanship of the factory the rest is a matter of choice and taste.

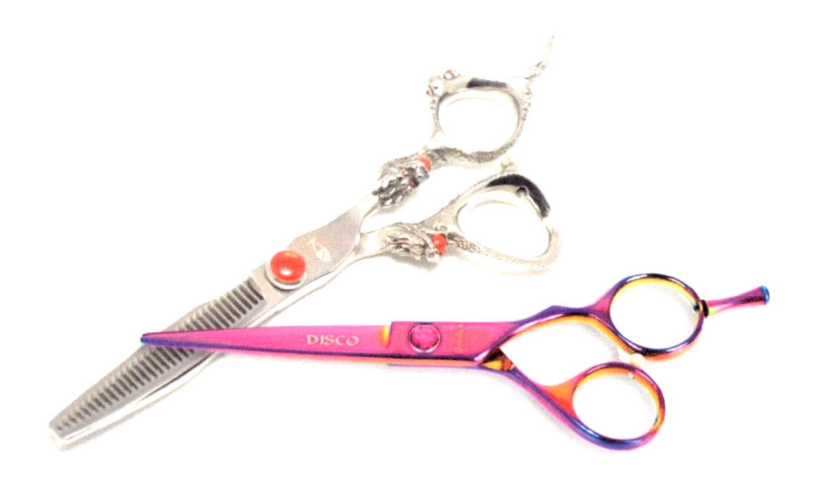

A good pair of shears will cost you $100.00 or more. The average shear purchased by hair stylists in the USA are around $200.00. Some companies are marketing much more expensive shears letting stylists make payments. When purchasing shears ask questions about the specifics of the steel and the country or origin. Get details on the warranty. We have encountered many high-pressure salesmen making large commissions who have intimidated young stylists into expensive shear purchases. Be a wise consumer when it comes to shopping for the main tool of your business.

The name brand of a shear is not always an indicator of quality. There are many knock-offs and imitation shears on the market. Many of the internet sites sell name brand shears that are not genuine. One of my clients bought a pair of these shears because it had a beautiful handle. She gave it to me to sharpen thinking I could make it cut like an expensive shear. I was able to improve the shear's cut, but it will never cut well because the workmanship and the steel were of such poor quality. Always purchase shears from an authorized dealer. The lists of authorized dealers can be found on the website of the manufacturer.

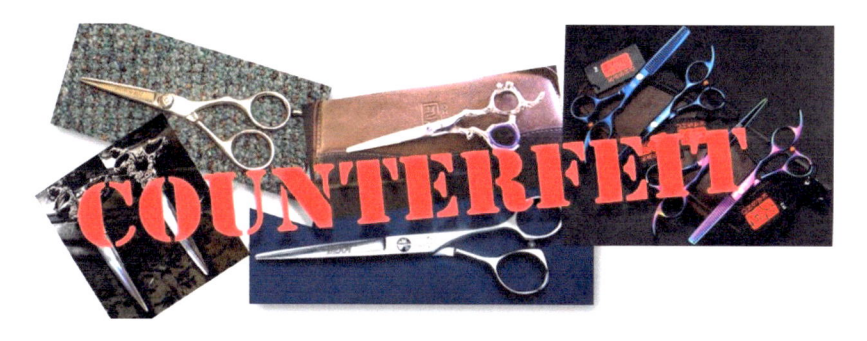

In addition to knock-off shears, some companies will have names very similar to expensive shears but not the same quality. The name may vary by only one letter. If you find a brand of shears that have a nice quality and fit your style of cutting, stay with that brand and that salesperson. This helps you build a rapport with your shears distributor and you will be buying tools you can rely on.

The shear length in most countries is measured by the length of the shear from the tip to the end, not including the finger rest. Some of the factories in Germany measures the length from the tip to the end including the finger rest UNLESS the finger rest is removeable. If the finger rest is removeable then the measurement does not include the finger rest. Therefore the same shear, the same size will be two different lengths in many German style shears if one has a fixed finger rest and the other has a removeable finger rest.

For example the two shears shown here would both measure as an 8" shear in the USA but the measurement on the top shear would be 8" and the bottom shear would be 8 ½" in Germany.

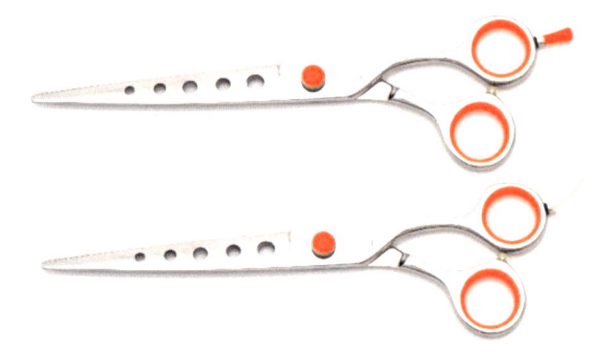

3
RUNNING WITH SHEARS

It is inevitable that all stylists will cut themselves. There are many reasons for cutting yourself all kinds of advice on how to prevent it. As mom said, *Don't run with scissors*.

The main reason stylists cut themselves is the shears are the wrong length for your hand. If your shears are too long or too short you are more apt to cut yourself. The blade of the shear that you use the most should be roughly the length of your longest finger. If you place the thumb hole next to the fleshy part of the palm of your hand and lay the shears in your hand the tip should fall in the section of the top digit of your *traffic* finger. (This is the long middle finger which is most often waved at my husband when he pulls out in front of someone in traffic). A great stylist will have shears longer and shorter than this for special purposes but will most commonly pick up the shear that fits their hand for their general cutting.

When a shear is too short, you tend to cut your knuckle. When a shear is too long you tend to cut in the web area between your fingers. Usually you will cut yourself more with a five-inch shear than one that is seven inches or longer.

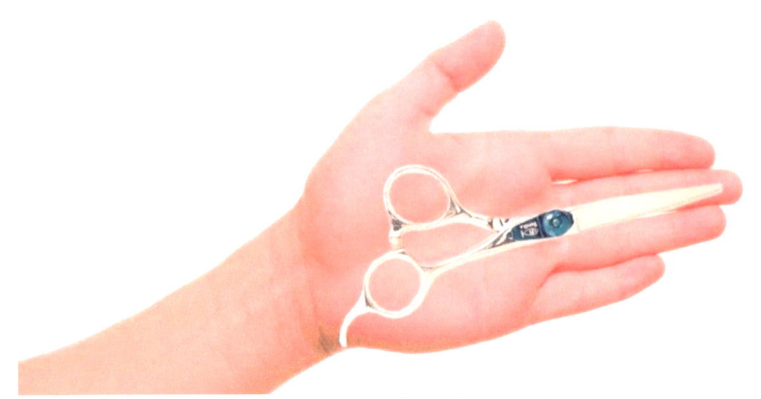

The shear you use the most should fit your hand.

> **DIY Idea:** If you have a habit of cutting your knuckle, wear a large ring on your middle finger of your left hand. (right for leftys) It will help protect your finger and give you a visual que where to stop cutting. Always remember when point cutting, close your shears as you are pulling out, not when you are coming into the hair.

Wear rings to protect your knuckles.

Another reason to cut yourself is picking the shears up incorrectly. If you pick up your shears, pick them up by the handle. If you pass a pair of shears to another person, hold the blades of the closed shears in your hand and point the handle to the next person. If the blades overlap and cut your hand while holding the blades, this may be due to a missing bumper or bent handle. Refer to the chapters on correcting bumpers to see how to fix this.

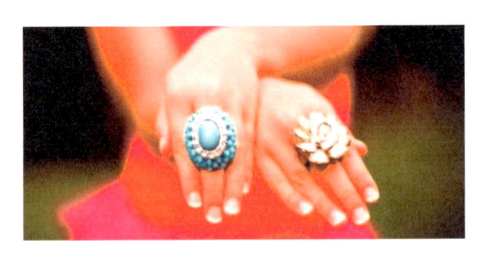

If you drop your shears, let your shears fall. Do not try to catch them with your hand or your foot. It is cheaper to have a pair of shears sharpened professionally than for you to miss work with a trip to the emergency room. A rubber mat on the floor under the chair will do more than comfort your feet. It will soften the blow if you drop your shears.

> **DIY Idea: If you happen to drop your shears and they land opened, the two blades may have nicked each other. Carefully pick them up without closing them. With your left hand (opposite if you are a left-handed person with lefthanded shears) spread the blades apart while you close the shear with your right hand. Let the shear close completely without the blades touching. Now slowly open the shears feeling for any catches or nicks.**
>
> **Repeat this process at least once or twice more. Then close the shears on a clean tissue using normal pressure. This process will push the nick to the outside of the blade instead of the inside. A nick on the outside is less damaging to the shears and you may be able to continue to use the shears without a problem. If the shears catch and will not close, don't try to cut with them. Contact your sharpener or follow the instructions in the chapter on edges.**

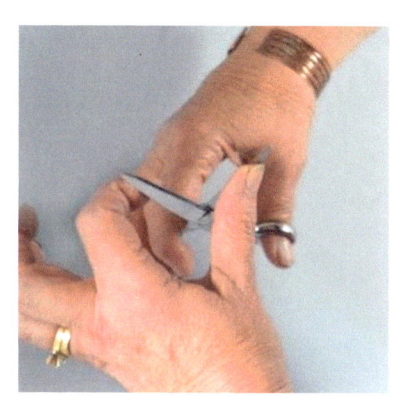

Before closing a shear after dropping, carefully push the blades apart to minimize nicks.

Usually when you drop shears, they will land in a partially open position. This will often create a nick on both blades where they touched. Sometimes they will land closed or completely open which will most likely cause little or no damage. A shear that hits point down or hits something hard as it falls can create an alignment problem. The shears may have sections of the blade, typically near the tip, that will not cut. This is a problem that is difficult for even a sharpener to fix.

Over the years there have been many designs and devices to prevent stylist from cutting their fingers or dropping their shears. I don't think any of them were very effective and probably were more dangerous than helpful.

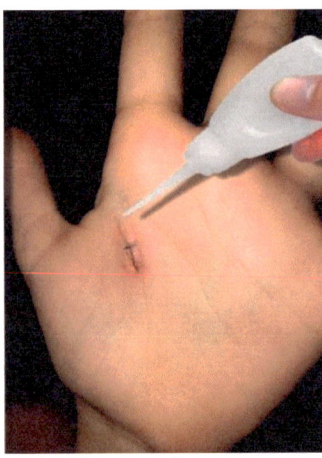

Applying super glue to a cut.

DIY Idea: If you have a minor cut on your hand or finger in a place too hard to bandage, use superglue to close the wound. It will keep it clean, hold up in water and even have less scarring than a regular plastic bandage. Superglue is cyanoacrylate. It is used in the medical profession in a variety of ways especially in skin grafts and plastic surgery. No superglue? Steal some nail glue from the manicurist station. Check the ingredient list. It is most likely cyanoacrylate.

4
DON'T HAVE A LOOSE SCREW!

If you stop reading after this chapter, you will have learned the most important DIY tool in your arsenal --- the correct adjustment of your shears. This is a DIY chore you MUST know because it will save you hundreds of dollars throughout the years. If a screw is too tight, you will work your hand too hard and the blades will wear incorrectly causing the shears to need sharpening more often. However, if you notice any of the following happen, you may have a loose screw. Don't be one of those stylists!

- Hair will flip or fold when you cut
- Hair will push
- Your hand will cramp as you apply side pressure to make the shears close properly
- Your blades will dull out and even nick
- Hair and debris will accumulate under the screw
- Your shears will wear out quicker and need replacing
- The cut will not be clean creating split ends on your client
- Your cuts will not be straight but will look like an upside down U shape
- Parts under the screw may shift so that the pivot is damaged
- Just like children, your shears will not behave because you have been too slack with them

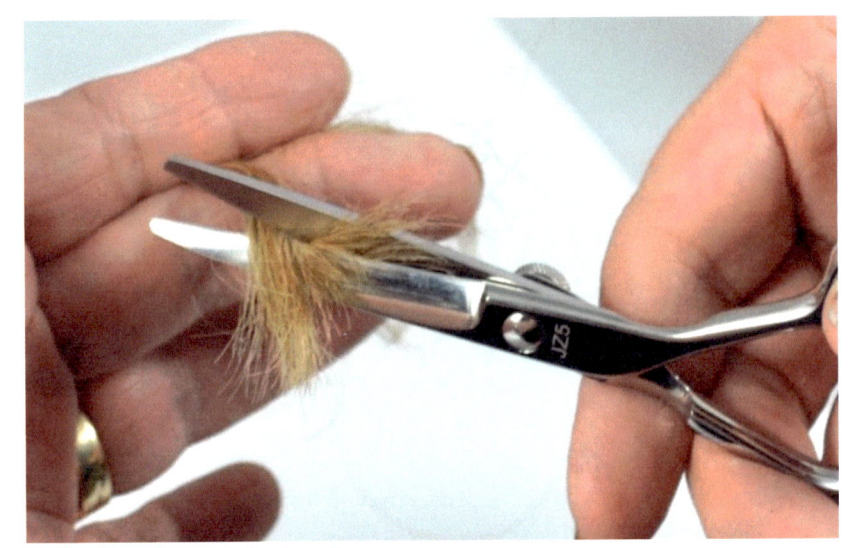

Hair flipping when cut due to a loose screw.

When I go into any typical hair salon, at least half of the shears in the salon will be too loose. Why is this? Number one is because the opening and closing causes things to shift and loosen, (the second law of thermodynamics, the law of entropy). The second reason is, stylist themselves will loosen the screw thinking this will make it easier on their hands when in fact their hands will work harder.

I was able to test correct shear adjustment scientifically using a knife sharpener tester. While teaching at a sharpening convention I encountered a device that measures the pressure it takes for a knife to penetrate a tomato peel. When I substituted a shear for a knife and a Puff tissue for a tomato I was able to obtain cut pressure measurements. I used only the tightness of the screw as the variable. The blade that swung freely, halfway closed, without slamming shut required the least pressure in cutting through the tissue.

So, what is the correct adjustment?

For MOST stylist shears the correct adjustment is where the shears will open and close freely without flopping. I generally tell my sharpeners and stylists to hold the shears facing you, perpendicular to the floor with the tip up and the handle down. Now holding the side of the finger hole which is the side that generally has the tang with your left hand, (this is all backwards for you leftys with lefty shears!) open the shears so that they form a cross or are at right angles to each other.

Next drop the thumb hole side of the handle that you are holding in your right hand. Let it swing freely down. If your shears are adjusted correctly this should close partially but not close completely. It should stay open to about $1/3^{rd}$ to $2/3^{rd}$ of the blade.

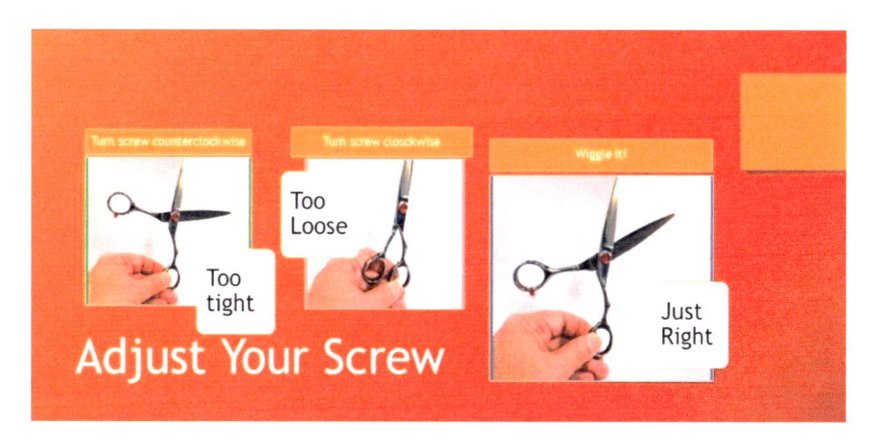

Adjust Your Screw

Turn screw counterclockwise — Too tight

Turn screw clockwise — Too Loose

Wiggle it! — Just Right

If the shears slam closed, your shears are too loose and need to be tightened. Tighten them a little at a time and check. I like to adjust them until the blades do not move at all then loosen them one click from that point. Since screws will tend to loosen with use, I personally like to adjust shears on the tight side, but that is my personal preference. Some shear manufacturers suggest that shears should be correctly adjusted just at the point where the blades don't move. Others want the screw so loose that it stops just short of closing all the way. My experiments with screw adjustments indicate that the one click looser causes the least pressure on the hand when closing them.

If the shears are too tight the shears will not close at all. Turn the screw to the left in the direction you would unscrew a lightbulb. Make a small turn.

Many screw types will have an audible click. If so, turn one click and check it. If your type of screw does not *click* turn it with what would be the

> **DIY Idea: Sometimes there seems to be no in-between. One click is too tight and will not move and the next is too loose. If this is the case, tighten the screw to one click to the over-tight adjustment. At this point, with the BLADES COMPLETELY OPEN (if the blades are touching, they will nick doing this), hold the handles with your two hands and wiggle it. Hold the left side of the handle (the thumb hole side) steady with your left hand and move your right hand holding the right side of the handle (the finger hole side) up and down as if you were shaking someone's hand. This will let the washer seat into place and loosen the screw. Now check the adjustment. In most cases the screw will be loosened and may even need to be tightened at this point.**

equivalent of 2 – 5 minutes on the face of a clock going counterclockwise.

Wiggle the handle on your shears to be sure the parts under the screw is seated correctly.

It is a wise precaution to check the adjustment of your shears each morning before you begin to cut. The salon fairies may have invaded your station and did nefarious things to your shears overnight. An inspection of your shears before your first hair cut each day is like a pilot inspecting his airplane. Don't start your day with a loose screw.

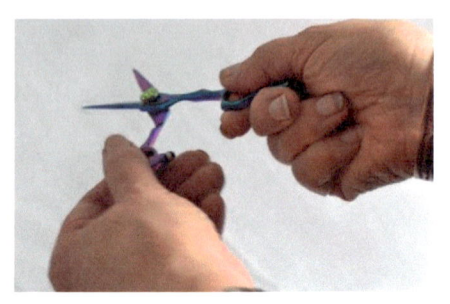

There are some exceptions to the rules on screw adjustment. Some shears with very thin light blades may need to be adjusted tighter. The weight of the blade compared to the heaviness of the handle makes the usual method of adjustment incorrect.

Another exception are shears with a ball bearing screw. These can and should be adjusted looser. They should not slam all the way closed but they do not need to be as tight. They will usually hold their adjustment better since there are no plastic washers inside under the screw head. Instead, there are many little stainless-steel balls inside a ring. You can sometimes recognize these types of screws without taking them apart because there is an additional ring with ball bearings around the screw head.

The Three Most Common Pivot Screw and How to Adjust Them

There are three most common screws: the thumb-nut screw, the regular screw and the UFO screw.

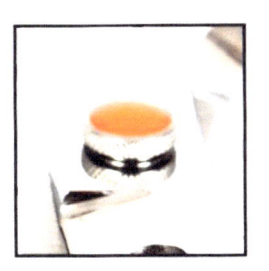

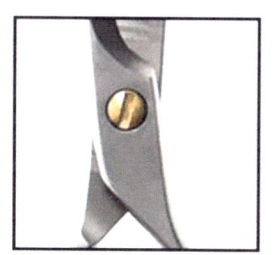

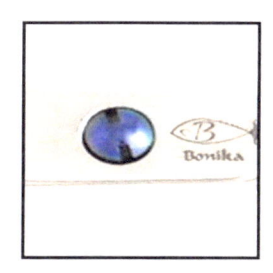

Left to right: The thumb nut screw, the regular screw and the UFO screw

DIY Idea: If you can't turn the thumb screw with your fingers and don't have pliers, grab it with the Gator Clip hair clip to give yourself extra

The **thumb nut screw** is the easiest to adjust. In most cases you will simply need to turn it using your thumb and forefinger. If it is tight or shallow so that it is hard to grip you can turn it with needle nose pliers.

The ***regular screw*** can be adjusted with a normal slotted screwdriver. These screws are less common than they were a few decades ago. Older shears are more likely to have these screws.

Some regular screws will look like there is a tiny screw on the back side of the shear with a larger slotted screw on the front. Don't be fooled. These are called split screws. You are seeing the split, not a tiny screw on the back. The shaft of the screw is split for the bolt of the screw to spread out and create a tighter connection. In reality, the split screw often gets mashed together so that the screw will not stay tight. This is a photo of s split screw with the shears taken apart.

> **DIY Idea: No screwdriver? Use a coin. A quarter will fit nicely into many screws. Some will need something thinner like a dime. If you can't get the screw to turn, soak the screw in oil or a product like Break Free™.**

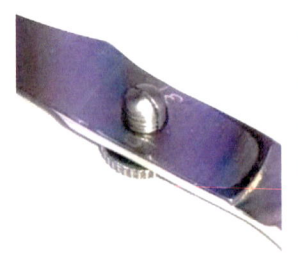

Split screw example

> **DIY Idea: Wrap Teflon™ or plumbers tape around the screw and reinsert it to hold the screw tighter. Never permanently glue the screw in. Loctite Blue™ or VibraTite VC-3™ are two other non-permanent bonding products that will also hold the screw in place yet will allow you to remove the screw later if needed.**

If this happens it is best to contact the manufacturer or distributor of the shears. Many companies cover this in the warranty. In some cases, like the Bonika Shears™ brand, you will not need your warranty card or receipt in order to get a warranty repair or replacement.

If it is not covered, take the screw out and try to widen the slot in the bolt. This can be done with a razor blade or extra thin screwdriver. Do this with the screw still inside one half of the shear as in the photo. Keep in mind the screw may break.

> **DIY Idea: No Loctite™ or Teflon tape™? Use double sticky tape or clear nail polish to hold your shear in place. You can also put a rubber band, weave thread or even a broom straw into the hole and reinsert the screw. The extra thickness may hold the screw in place.**

A safer approach would be to rough up the threads on the screw by raking your screwdriver over the threads of the screw. This will create a slight damage to the threads with burs that will catch, and make the screw less apt to back out.

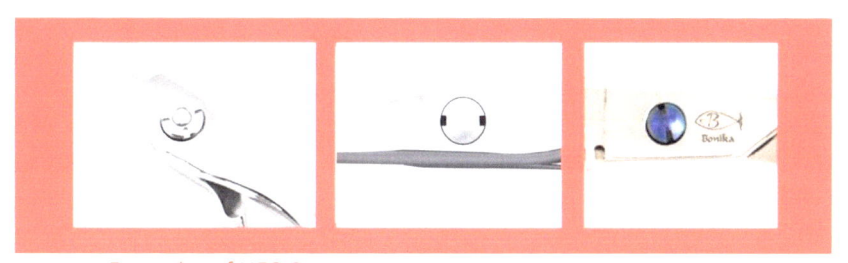

Examples of UFO Screws

Some screws on stylist shears are very strange looking. These don't have a slot. Instead there are two little slits or holes that look like snake-eyes. Sometimes they even have 4 slots. An employee of Bonika Shears began calling these **UFO Screws** when they first appeared on shears. The term became the colloquial word for these screws in the USA and many other countries. Officially they are called *tamper resistant screws* although different manufacturers will have other names for them. These are the best screws at this time for holding their adjustment because they are not easily loosened. Like the thumb-nut screw, they are composed of many little parts often including an internal clicker plate.

To tighten or loosen this nut you will need a special made *shear key* or *ufo tool*. These come in a variety of shapes and are normally included with your shear purchase. To use this tool, find the spines with spacing to match the holes in your screw. Insert the spines into the holes and turn the screw to either tighten or loosen.

Hardware stores sell screwdriver bits called *spanner bits* that may fit the holes in your particular pair of stylist shears. Many manufacturers and sharpeners will modify a screw driver with a Dremel™ tool to make their own tool for adjusting these shears. These home-made tools made from screwdrivers are popular because it is hard to get a grip on the tiny screw keys that come with the shears. The tools can be grabbed with a vise-grip or inserted into a slot cut into a dowel stick for extra torque.

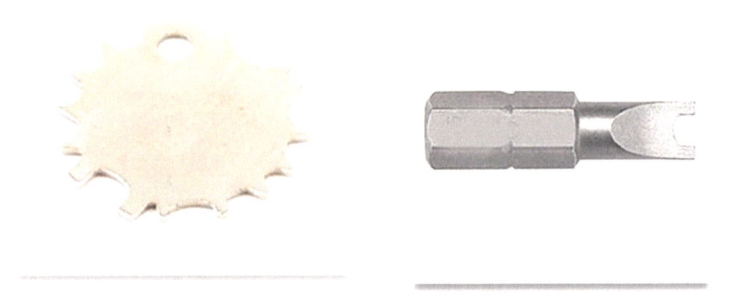

Typical UFO tool or screw key and a spanner bit

Just like the other screws, if this screw seems defective it is most likely covered under the warranty from your manufacturer. These screws have very few problems unless a part inside the screw is lost or broken.

Adjusting the screws of your beauty shears is the most important care and maintenance skill you can have. It will save you money and frustration to keep your screws properly set.

In Atlanta, our office and sharpening training facility is located on the eastern section of the metropolitan area. To drive across the city with the intense traffic can be very maddening and time consuming. One afternoon a stylist drove two hours through the middle of Atlanta to reach our office because she thought her shears were so dull, she could not work the next day. We took one quick look at them. We tighten the screw. We let her test them and cut with them and they worked perfectly. I can't repeat what she said but she was very angry with herself. We did not charge her, but she gave us a big tip for being honest about her cutting tools.

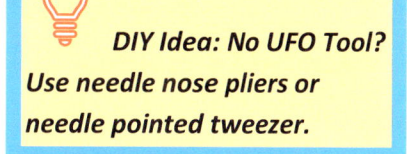

> **DIY Idea: No UFO Tool?**
> **Use needle nose pliers or needle pointed tweezer.**

This similar scenario has been repeated at our office many times. Before you send your shears off for sharpening or call a sharpener, check the tension of your screw.

Two exceptions to the rule on the tension on your screw is a ball bearing screw and the Firefly screw. Shears with a ball bearing type structure can often function with a looser tension while shears with slender light blades and small pivot area like the Firefly need a tighter tension.

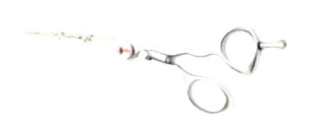

Firefly shear with slender blades needs to be adjusted tighter.

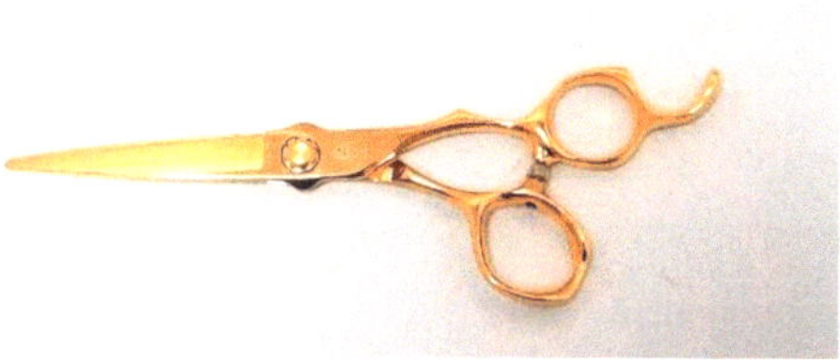

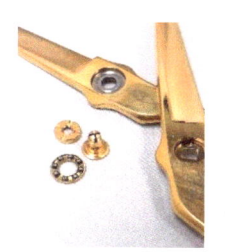

Shears with ball bearing type screws hold their adjustment better and may not need to have as tight of tension.

5
HOW TO CLEAN AND DISINFECT YOUR SHEARS

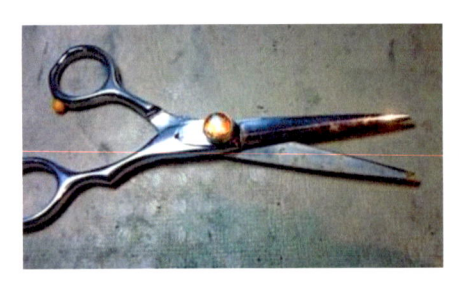

There are two reasons to clean your shears. Number one is hygiene. In most areas the government mandates that cutting tools be kept clean so as not to spread diseases. The other reason to keep your shears clean is to prevent rust. Most modern stylist shears have chromium added as an alloy to the steel. Steel with at least 10.5% chromium is called *stainless steel* or *inox steel*. Chromium makes the steel harder and tougher, but it also helps prevent tarnish and rust. Chromium can only do its job if it comes in contact with oxygen. Shears that are kept dirty prevent oxygen from reaching the steel and they will rust. I have seen terrible examples of shears rusting and pitting because they were left dirty. Keeping your shears clean will not only make you compliant with the ordinances of your area, but it will save you money in sharpening bills and shear replacements.

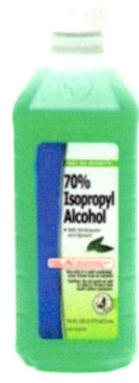

My number one recommendation for cleaning shears is isopropyl alcohol also known as rubbing alcohol. 70% alcohol is the strength of choice. The lower percentage has more water and is harsher on the shears. A higher percentage strangely enough is less effective in killing bacteria and viruses. The higher concentration of water keeps the alcohol on the surface of the metal longer before it evaporates thereby making in more efficient as a disinfectant. It should be used in conjunction with some agitation, using, in my opinion, a microfiber cloth.

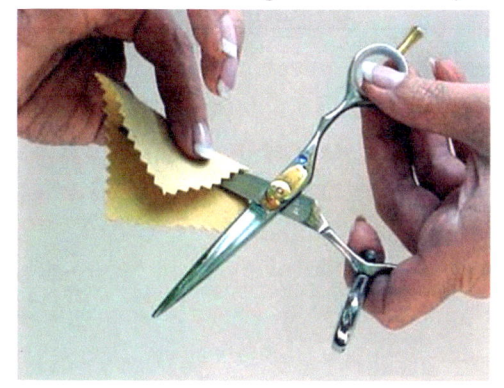

Always wipe with the non-sharp side next to your hand.

Wet the cloth with the alcohol and wipe the blade with the spine facing the palm of your hand. Be sure your fingers or thumb do not slide over the edge of the blade. Even with the thick cloth the blade is sharp enough it can cut through right to your fingers.

> **DIY Idea: No alcohol? Use hand sanitizer followed by a damp cloth to remove any sticky residue.**

Most of the spray disinfectants have a lot of water in them. Sometimes Other methods of cleaning have their drawbacks. Barbicide™ type products are mostly water which can be tough on metals. Never dip your shears in these products so that the moisture gets under the screw. The moisture held there can cause rust.

Many stylists will think a quick spray from their aerosol canned disinfectant is enough to clean their blades. This is not a very green policy for the world and is not efficient for cleaning shears. Without wiping and adding some agitation this method will not kill all the germs and will not remove hair and products left behind. Hair and product on a blade can generate rust. However, there is one spray disinfectant I highly recommend. It is H-42™ which is an oil-based disinfectant. The shear blades must still be wiped before to remove any debris. I especially like this product since it was invented by a chemist here in my town of Atlanta. It is good for the metal, inhibits rust, smells good and is 99.9% effective against viruses and bacteria. It is the perfect product for your clippers as well. We sell this on line at Bonika.com or you can buy it in most countries of the world in stores that sell barber supplies.

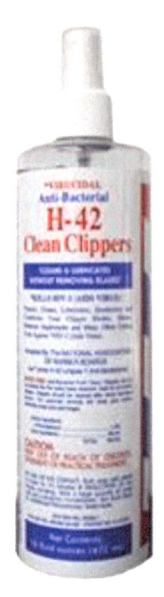

When you wipe your shear blades don't use paper towels or terry cloth towels. These can be harsh on the sharp blade edge. Use a soft cloth to wipe your shears to preserve the sharpness of your edge. Many shears will come with a soft leather chamois. This is a great item to wipe your shears and protect the edge. However, my product of choice to wipe shears is still a microfiber cloth.

> *DIY Idea: Are your shears gummy from dried on product or weave glue? Nail polish remover will clean off the gunk. It is also a disinfectant of sorts, although it is not as effective as other products. I suggest you follow this with either the isopropyl alcohol or H42™.*

A quick wipe with alcohol between clients is an advisable practice then give your shears a thorough clean at the end of the day.

> **DIY Idea: Dental floss and a toothbrush can clean the pivot area of the shear. Work the hair from between the blades without removing the screw by using your dental floss. Brush hair and debris away with the toothbrush.**

I find that stylists will shop for pretty shears with rhinestones or colors or fancy handles. Clients notice if you have expensive looking shears. They also notice if your shears are dirty and covered with dried on product or hair. Keeping on top of cleaning your shears quickly between clients and thoroughly cleaning at the end of the day will keep your shears gleaming. This will impress your clients and will keep your edges sharper longer.

6

HOW TO FIGHT RUST AND KEEP THE SHINE

There might be hair on the floor around your station. You may have on your counter the residues of the sandwich from the restaurant next door. You might even have hair color on the towel draped over your chair and hair in your comb. Those items may bring a fine with the State Board but they will still cost you less money than leaving your shears dirty.

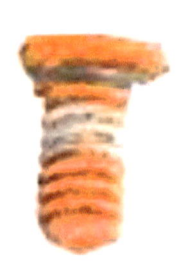

As stated before, a dirty shear very quickly becomes a rusty shear. A shear with a rusty pivot screw and blades will need sharpening and may have to be replaced. The most dangerous place for rust to form is inside the pivot screw. Rust on the outside of the blade can be removed but rust in the threads of the screw hole cannot be repaired. Once the threads inside the shear rust out, there is very little that can be done to keep the correct adjustment for the blades.

Refer to the previous chapter on how to properly clean your shears. Give them a thorough cleaning at the end of each day, then it is time to oil your shears.

> **DIY Idea – Rust forming on your shears?** Remove rust using an ordinary pencil. Both the eraser and the pencil lead itself work well in rust removal. An everyday eraser will take off most rust. If the rust is deeper, use the lead of the pencil. Graphite is harder than rust but softer than steel. It will scratch off the rust without scratching the metal underneath.

Most stylists never oil their shears. I was on stage at a large international hair show in Las Vegas and I asked the stylists in the room who oils their shears. With about 200 professional and student stylists there, only two raised their hand. Very few stylists oil their shears or even know how to oil their shears. Any time you have metal rubbing against metal, especially in the presence of water, oil is important.

Oil shears at the pivot area where the blades touch.

At the end of each day, after you have cleaned your shears and before you safely put them away, oil the halfmoon area behind the pivot screw of your shears. Oiling your shears is like brushing your teeth each night. It will make you a lot more pleasant in the morning and will preserve your health and your wallet.

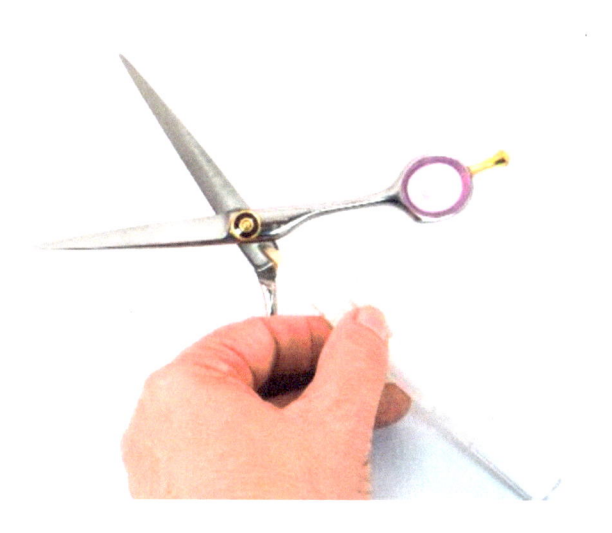

Most shear manufacturers recommend high-quality Camilla oil. This is a Japanese oil used for centuries on swords, cutlery and even cosmetics.

Many stylists use clipper oil. Clipper oil is better than no oil at all, but it is a little too thick and sticky. Sewing machine oil and gun oil are also products that are effective in keeping your shears working well. WD-40™ and H42™ are acceptable but are thinner than Camilla oil and do not work as well.

> **DIY Idea** – For an incredibly smooth cut and great protection from rust, use lip balm.
>
> This idea came from South Carolina sharpener Jim Turner. I generally suggest Burt's Bees™ or a good quality lip balm that is simply wax and oil. Open the shears and run the stick over the halfmoon area behind the pivot and along the edges of the shears. The wax fills in any small grind marks and the oil lets the blades glide over each other. Wipe off the excess with a soft tissue. This can be done daily. The lip balm trick helped me place first in the sharpening certification. The smooth feel is unlike anything you have tried.

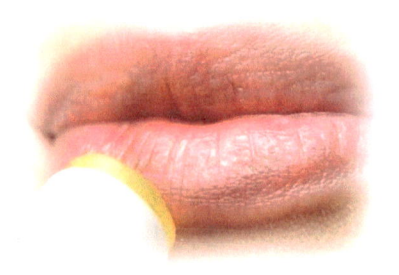

Apply a quality lip balm with wax and oil to the edge of your shears and at the pivot area. Wipe off excess.

Do you want an extra shiny shine? Use a jeweler's cloth. These cloths have chemicals embedded in the fabric and will bring an extra luster in shine to your shears. This in turn will help in inhibiting rust. Just as the elements will dull the finish on a fine automobile, neglect in the care of your shears will lead to not only a dulling of the shine but the dulling of the edge. Jeweler's cloths can be purchased at any place that sells jewelry. You may already have one. If you decide to use any of the harsh compounds like chrome polish be careful not to get it on the edge and clean the shears thoroughly with isopropyl alcohol before you close the blades. It is best not to use any chemicals stronger than a jeweler's cloth to clean your blades.

If acid or other harsh chemicals fall on your shears, your sharpener may be able to buff it off. Sometimes acid from our own bodies will turn the handles of the shears a tarnished gray. In these cases, even if the shears were buffed up, your body chemistry will bring the tarnish back. This would be a good opportunity to replace your shears with one of the PVD or titanium coated colored shears.

The colored coated shears have their own set of problems. If the color comes off, there is no safe way to put the color back on. Safe, that is for the shears. All the coatings and colors have a heat element involved in the process which can damage the strength of the steel. These would need to be replaced or used as is with their beauty marred.

7
WHERE TO HOUSE YOUR SHEARS

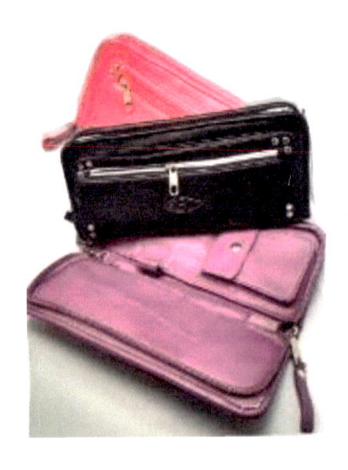

Your shears are your money-making babies. They need a good home and a *car seat* when you travel with them. The best place for your shears to live is in a nice leather case or pouch. It should be able to snap them in securely, so they won't drop. The leather allows the shears to breathe. This allows the chromium alloy in the stainless steel to combine with oxygen to protect your shears from rust.

However, the State Board of Cosmetology in our state of Georgia wants the *clean* shears when not in use to be put in a closed container. This can't be leather because they want something that can be completely disinfected and cleaned of hair. It is always a compromise.

There are some places where you do not want to put your shears. They are as follows:

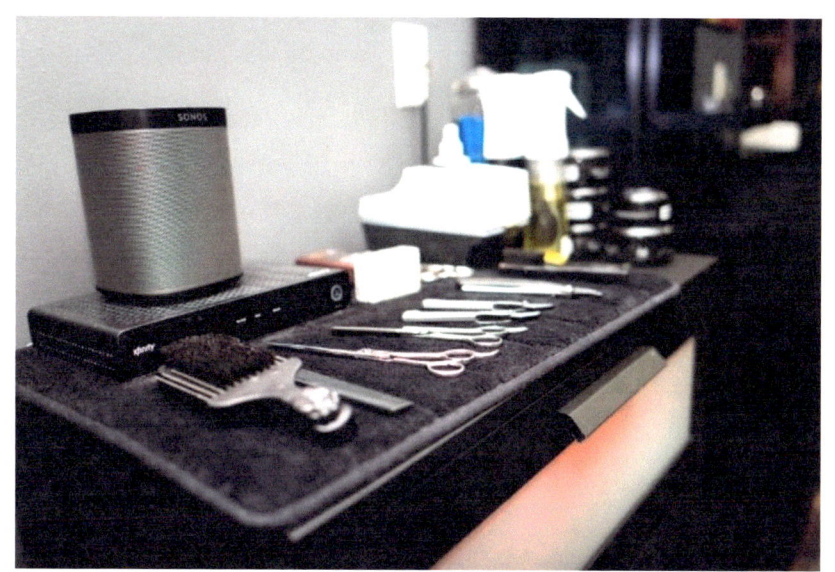

Typical layout of shears during the day which is required by many USA State Boards. This is not the safest way to display your shears because clients are tempted to pick them up.

Don't leave your shears out on your station laying on a towel. When your back is turned your client may pick them up and cut a tag off their new blouse, tighten a loose screw on your station, play with the adjustment screw like a musical instrument or hand them to their child to cut paper dolls out of the salon magazines. Your shop manager can accidently pick them up along with your terry cloth towels and put them in the washing machine. A bored child can pick them up and cut through your clipper cord. The manicurist whom you made angry by stealing her yogurt from the refrigerator can grab them and run her nail file down the edge. All of these are situations I have encountered as emergency repair calls. Any of these things can happen in an instant while your back is turned mixing color.

Don't throw them in a drawer with everything else. Shears loose in a drawer can hit other shears and get nicked; the tip can be damaged when they slide back and forth as you open and close the drawer. You can also cut yourself badly as you reach into the drawer to retrieve them.

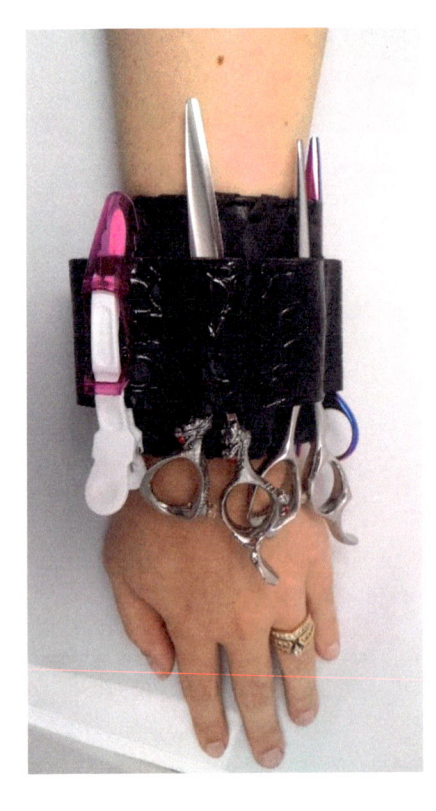

Example of one of many unusual shear carriers. Be cautious that any tool belt or strap holds your shears securely.

Don't put them back into the little plastic zippered case. Sometimes new shears will come in a clear plastic case that closes tightly. If there is any dampness on the shears the case will act as a sauna, especially if you leave them in the car and they can rust. If you want to use this case just for quick transportation home or to a client's location, this is acceptable, but long-term storage and overnight storage is not good unless you are certain the shears are dry.

Don't hang them on the rack attached *to your stove irons.* I know there are slots on some of the irons that are designed to hold shears, but the heat from the irons can cause the rubber bumpers and the plastic washers to crack. If you find you are always having to have your bumpers replaced, check to see if your storage area is near dry heat.

Don't hang your shears on a magnetic rack. Strips of strong magnetics are sold to hang shears and other tools. The magnetic strength that is strong enough to hold a shear is also strong enough to magnetize the shear. Be careful if you use one of the magnetic wrist bands that hold shears. Long term exposure to magnets can cause metal dust particles to collect on the steel and grime accumulates. The other problem with using magnets is that the shears are not as secure and can fall more easily.

Find a safe dry place to store your shears away from extreme heat. Air should reach them even though state regulations often require an airtight container. Never immerse them in water or a water mixture. The case you use should be cleanable. You should be able to blow out any hair with the cool setting of your hair dryer and wipe it clean of debris. Your cloth with isopropyl alcohol will also work to clean and disinfect your shear case. When your shears are safely stored in the home of your choice, put them into your drawer or set to the back of your station away from the hands of your client.

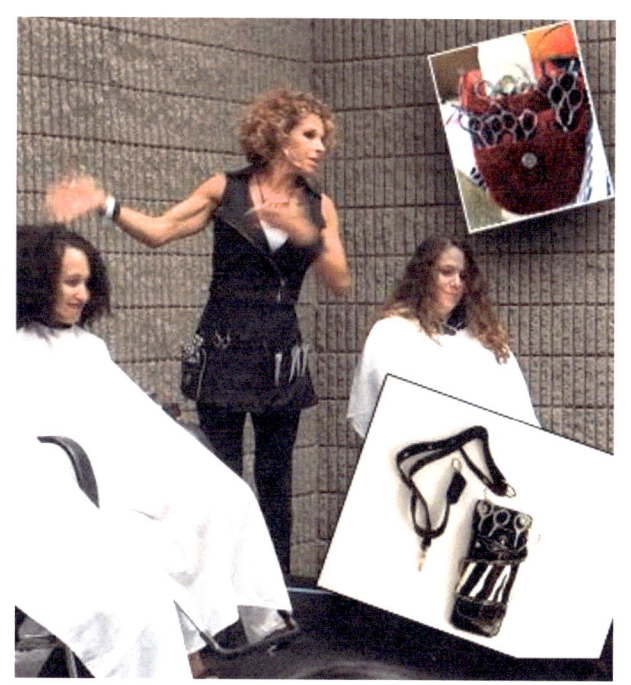

Examples of tool holsters and aprons. Pictured here, Christina Carsillo presenting on stage at the Bronner Brothers International Beauty Show wearing a tool apron.

Some shear companies now have a plastic bubble type case that is not only cleanable but protects your shears if they fall. These individual cases are a great innovation to help stylists. If your local regulatory agency will allow it use holsters, arm bands and aprons designed for holding your shears. This keeps your shears with you, gives you easy access to your shears and displays your collection so that your client can see that you are well equipped to give them a quality haircut.

> 💡 **DIY Idea: Plastic pencil cases work well since they have a lid, are easily cleaned and come in a variety of colors. Be sure to get a different box for each pair of shears since you don't want them banging against each other and nicking each other. If you must store two shears in one box have the handles in opposite directions to minimize nicks. These boxes are on sale during August and September.**

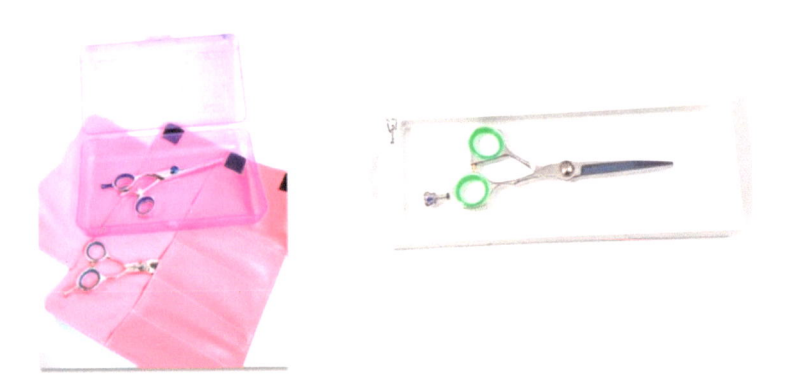

Left: A typical leatherette case for carrying shears compared to a pencil box. Right: Bubble type display packaging for shears.

When transporting your shears, a new level of secure storage is involved. Now it is good to use the clear plastic case or other case that came with your shears if practical. Be sure the shears are closed when you secure them. Close and snap your case. Never have shears loose in a purse or a pocket. This is not only dangerous for your shears but could involve a trip to the hospital for stitches for yourself.

If you are shipping your shears, a box is better than a bag, especially if you have curved shears. Cushioned bags are good enough, unless the shipper stacks a heavy box on your shears. This can affect the alignment. Always insure your shears and put your information inside the case with the shears as well as on the package.

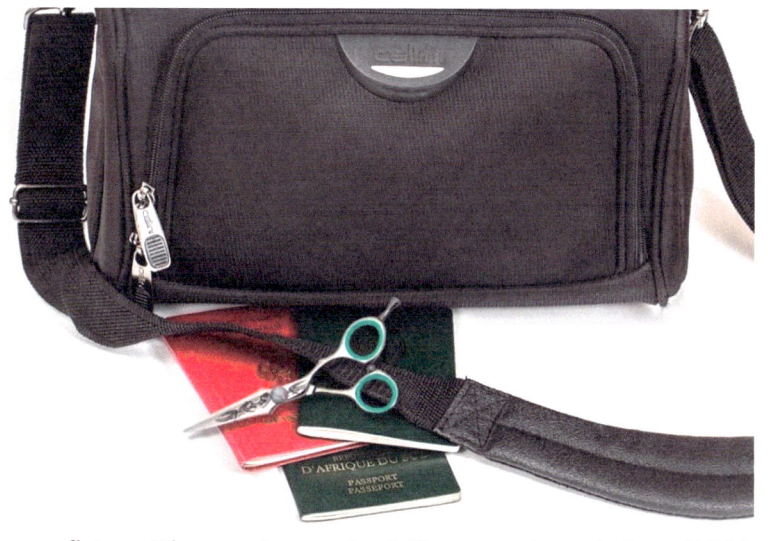

If you are flying with your shears, check the current regulations. Within the United States, most normal length stylist shears can now be put in carry-ons. As of this time any shear with a blade of 4 inches or less can be a carry-on item. Most 7-inch shears have a blade of less than 4 inches and will go through screening. As we all know the travel regulations vary, so check the latest before arriving at the airport.

DIY Idea - Secure the tip of your shears when transporting them for protection of yourself and your shears. You can use the soft tubing from a fish tank pump or a hospital IV tube. Cut a one-inch section and slide it over the tip for protection. A soft drinking straw will also work. So will a rubber band. Never tape your shears shut. The residue is hard to remove, and the tape can trap dampness and generate rust.

Twice this week I spoke

to women who were able to go through the Atlanta airport checkpoint with their shears, but they were confiscated when they entered an overseas airport checkpoint. Don't assume every airport is the same. To be safe, pack your shears in your luggage. If you have a lot of expensive shears, insure them. There have been instances when stylists have reported them stolen out of their suitcases.

> *DIY Idea - Use twist ties from a bread bag to tie around the handles of the blade to keep the shears closed when transporting. No twist ties? Tie a bow with a colorful hair ribbon!*

8
HOW TO REPLACE FINGER RESTS

Not everyone likes a finger rest on their shears. I've found some stylists; especially European trained stylists, prefer to cut with shears without finger rests. This is why many shears have removeable finger rests. At this time the more popular shears have a fixed finger rest that is permanently attached. If these finger rests break off there is no alternative but to solder one back on. This rarely happens. The detachable finger rests, however, have problems all the time. They are always coming off.

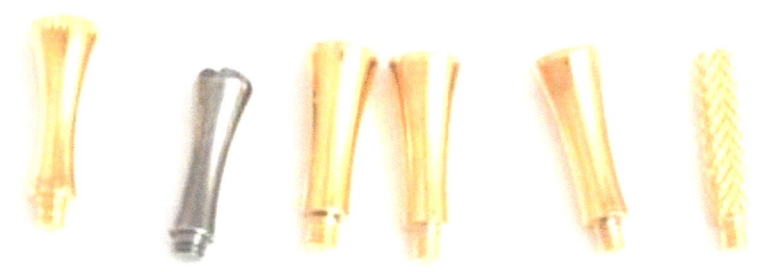

If your finger rest comes off and you have not lost it, you can simply screw it back on. If you are a stylist who likes to rest their pinky on the finger rest and you have a screw-on finger rest and the finger rest comes off and gets lost, it can put a bummer on your day. If you have a finger rest with the tendency to come off, Loctite™, Gorilla Glue™ or any non-water-soluble super glue will hold the finger rest in place.

> **DIY Idea – No super glue for your finger rest? Use a drop of nail glue or nail polish on the threads of your finger rest and screw it back in. It will keep it in place.**

The hole for the finger rest is very small. Sometimes it was drilled improperly in the factory, either too large or at an angle. If the finger rest still wobbles after gluing it in, put weave thread or some thread inside the hole, then add glue to the threads and screw it in. The width of the thread will make the finger rest hold tighter and prevent the wobble.

How to Make a Finger Rest if Yours is Gone.

Solution 1: *Buy a bolt.* Go to the hardware store and find a small bolt that will fit in the hole of your finger rest. Typically, they will be 2.5, 2.8 or 3 mm thread. Cut part of a small plastic drinking straw a little shorter than the length of your bolt. Slide the straw over the bolt and screw into place. Use some non-permanent glue to hold it in place so you can replace it with a proper finger rest later.

Solution 2: *Buy a bag of watercolor brushes.* Purchase a bag of cheap children's water color paint brushes that come 12 for a dollar. Pick a color you like and glue the tip of the paint brush into the hole using nail glue or other quick set glue. Trim the brush end of the paint brush to the desired length.

Solution 3: *Have a scavenger hunt.* Find other items in your salon that will substitute for a finger rest. You can use an old rat tail comb, the cheaper the better and glue the tip into the space and cut to length. A toothpick if thick enough might work. Some salons have old curler picks that can work for a finger rest hack.

Below is an improvised finger rest using an old color brush. Put glue in the hole then push the tip through the hole. After the glue dries trip the length to the size finger rest you need with snips and trim out the inside flush with a razor blade or Exacto™ knife.

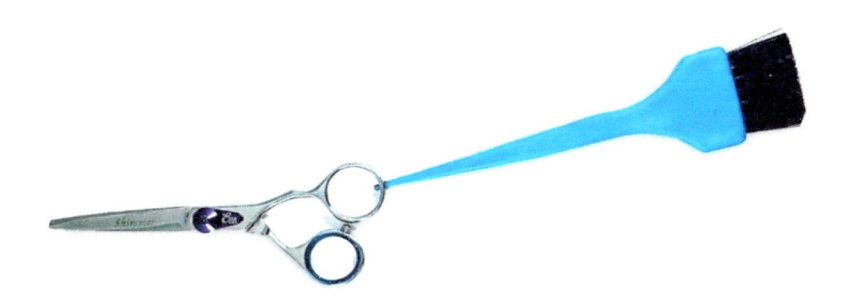

Glue in the brush tip. After glue dries snip the rest of the brush off to the desired finger rest length.

9
HOW TO REPLACE BUMPERS

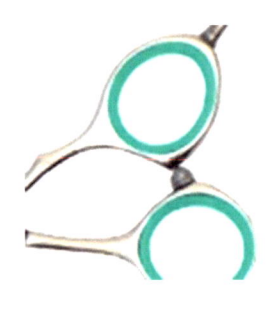

The bumper is the spacer between the handles of your shears. The purpose of it is to protect your hand from the harsh repetitive jarring motion of closing your shears over and over. Shears without bumpers can cause terrible permanent hand damage. These were a great innovation to the beauty industry.

In addition to cushioning your hand, the bumper also makes your shears quieter. Without it your shears would go click, click, click every time you close them. That is why it is also called a silencer. If you notice a clicking sound as you close your shears, your bumper may be gone.

More important than keeping your shears quiet, the bumper keeps the blades from overlapping. Without it the edge at the tip is exposed making it easy to cut yourself or your client. It also gets nicked easier. If you notice you are cutting yourself more, this could also indicate you have a missing bumper or a worn bumper. Sometimes a bumper breaks off or is worn down to the point the blades will overlap but the shears will be quiet because a small portion of the bumper is still there.

There are two common types of bumpers; the screw-in bumper and the pull through bumper. There are other bumpers on the market, but these are rare and may be best left to the professional sharpeners.

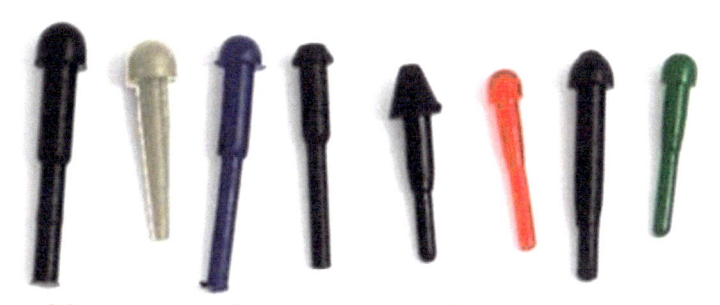

Pull-through bumpers come in many colors and sizes.

The *pull through bumpers* are the traditional type bumpers on Japanese style shears. They have a rubber head or ball and a long tail. These bumpers come in a variety of sizes and can be modified if too large by using a razor blade or Exacto™ knife to trim it to the hole. If you order pull-through bumpers, order several sizes (they are typically less than $1 each). You can order these online from Bonika.com.

New pull through bumpers are easy to install. First, remove any residue or debris or remnants of the current bumper. You might use a dental floss pick for this or pointed tweezers. Pull the tail of the bumper through the hole in the handle's finger hole. While pulling on the tail (you may need to use needle nose pliers for this) don't pull the head of the bumper flush to the metal. Stop just before pulling it all the way in and put a drop of glue on the neck of the bumper. One of the instant bonding glues work well for this. After that, pull it through the

DIY Idea – No super glue for your bumper? Use a drop of nail glue or nail polish on the neck of your bumper and pull it through. It will keep it in place.

rest of the way. Once you are sure the glue is dry, trim off the excess tail. Close the shears. If there is space between the blades at the tip, trim down the bumper so that there is a slight overlap of the blade.

> **DIY Idea – To be sure your bumper stays put, leave a little tail inside the finger hole. Light this with a lighter and use your needle nose pliers or other metal item to mash the melted bumper to make a plug on the inside of the hole in your finger hole. You can also melt the head of the bumper and close the shears to the right position to melt the head of the bumper to size.**

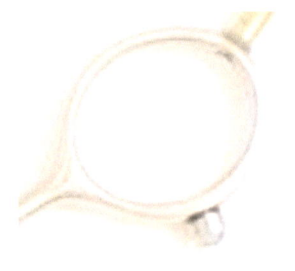

Screw-in bumper type

The other type of bumper is the screw-in bumper. The screw-in bumper is a screw with a plastic cap on top. If it is completely missing and you have this type of bumper, you will see threads inside the hole. Look around and see if you can find the lost bumper, if so, you can simply screw it back in. If it is missing, you will need to order another one. Once again you can order this from Bonika.com. They typically come in two sizes so order both sizes because you will not know what size you have. Loctite™ or other non-permanent glue may be used to keep the bumper in place.

Sometimes you will see the screw-in bumper still in place. Maybe it looks like a split screw head with remnants of plastic around it. The plastic can wear off the screw. These screw caps can be purchased from a company, like Bonika Shears, that sells scissor parts. Put a drop of glue on the head of the screw and push the cap on. Usually it is easier to replace the entire bumper. If you don't have a screw-in bumper, you can use a pull through bumper. You may have to trim the tail down skinnier to fit in the hole.

Often it is advisable to order a repair kit with assorted shear parts for emergencies. These kits like the one with the parts pictured here are also available on the Bonika website.

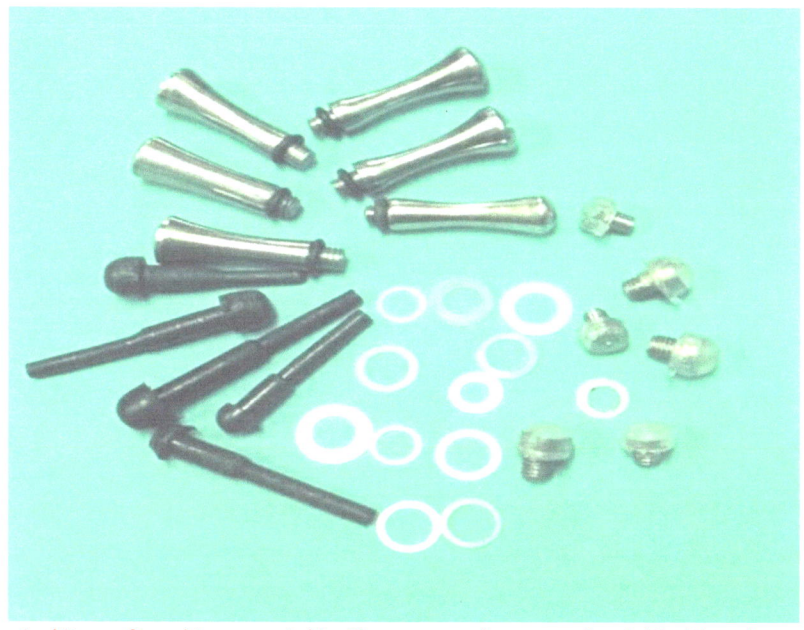

Typical items found in a repair kit. Finger rests, bumpers (both kinds) and assorted washers to go under the screw head.

What if you don't have any type of bumper and you must use your shears? I have seen many creative hacks for replacing bumpers over the years. You could use a rubber band tied around the finger hole. One stylist used the top off a ball point pen for a bumper. Other times I've

DIY Idea – If the plastic is worn off your screw-in bumper put a drop of glue from a hot glue gun on the screw head. Let it cool slightly so it is malleable but is secured into place. Close the shears so that the tips just cross over the rideline at the tip and let the glue finish cooling.

seen toothpicks and pieces of rubber wired on and even eyeglass nose pads. Be sure that when you call your sharpener to replace this part you use the right name. I've had an emergency call from a cosmetology school with a frantic teacher on the phone crying, "Help, all our *balls* have fallen off."

If you have a quality shear like a Bonika™ Shear and others, the bumpers may be covered under the lifetime warranty. If you know the shear model and call the manufacturer, they may simply drop the part in the mail to you at no charge. The easiest solution while you wait is to wrap a band-aid around the area so there is separation between the handles and cushion for your hand. This will suffice until your sharpener comes and can replace your bumper.

> ***DIY Idea - Replace the bumper with rubber perm curler replacements. The rubber rods can be removed from a curler, cut in half and put into the hole. Trim off the excess tail. Additional perm rod rubbers can be purchased from most beauty supplies.***

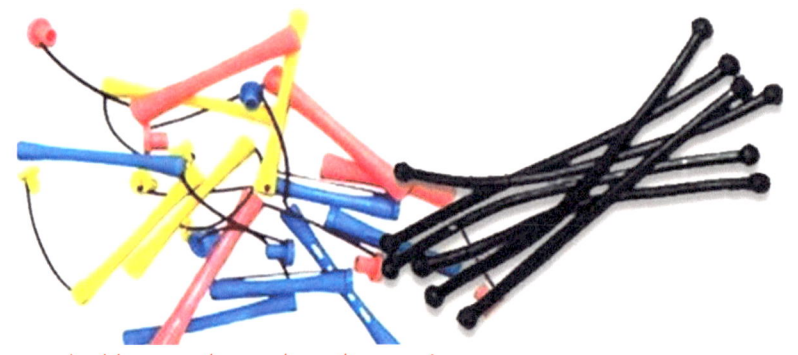

Perm rod rubbers can be used as a bumper in an emergency.

10
HOW TO MAKE YOUR SHEARS FIT YOUR FINGERS

Are your fingers too large for the finger holes of your shears? There is no DIY trick to fix that. However, there are ways to keep your finger and thumb from sliding in too far into the holes on the handle of your shears.

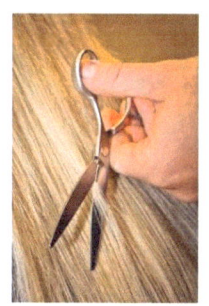

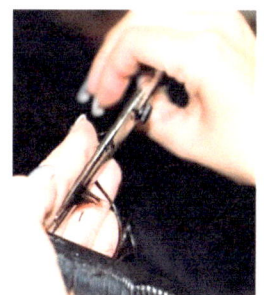

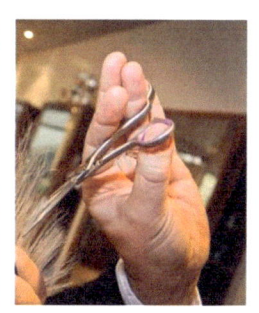

Three examples of correct hand positioning

If you hold your shears correctly like most cosmetology instructors and cutting experts teach, only the tip of your thumb is in the thumb hole and the ring finger should go into the finger hole only up to the first joint. The pinky finger stabilizes the hand by lying on the finger rest. Correct cutting means that only the thumb is moving, and the fingers stay relaxed and straight. This helps prevent carpal tunnel syndrome plus it allows your cut to be straighter. Shears are designed to be used in this manner. If the palm muscles open and close the shear because the thumb and finger are pushed too far inside the holes this can affect the life of the shear. The handle can be bent and no longer lineup correctly and the shears blades will come together at an odd angle. This positioning is called "side pressure" cutting or sometimes "crab grip" cutting. It is not good for the shears or your hand.

If your fingers are small and the thumb and finger holes are large it is hard to hold the shears in the correct way. Therefore, sizers or insert rings were invented. Some rings are a gummy plastic that gives a good grip and control of the shears. Other rings are a smooth hard plastic allowing the thumb to glide in and out of the thumb hole with less effort. You will need to decide what style is best for you. All will make the holes smaller and give a firmer, more stable grip.

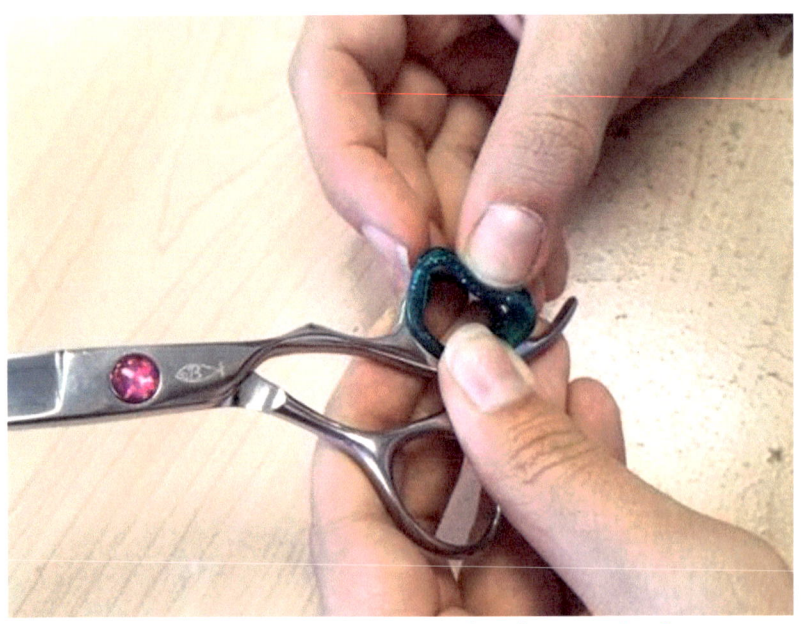

Inserting a ring into a shear. Sometimes it needs to be coaxed to fit.

Insert rings come in a variety of colors and sizes. The sizes are usually selected by the size of the holes on the shears, not the size of your fingers. It is my experience that quality hand sharpened shears may vary in the size of the finger rings needed from one shear to another, even though they are the same model. This is why it can be difficult to order rings for a shear without actually putting them into the shear holes themselves. If you are unable to purchase sizer rings without your shears present to fit them, it is often best to buy a few different sizes. Many of the companies that sell rings sell them in a 6-pack of three sizes of rings. Sometimes fingers are so small and the holes so large that the rings can be doubled with a ring inside a ring.

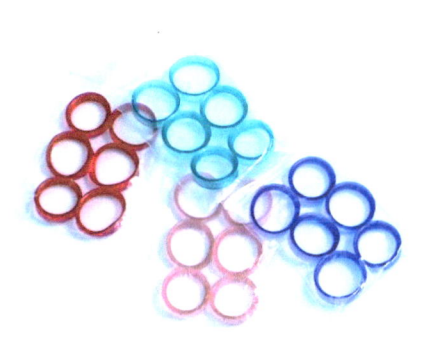

Examples of ring 6-packs

There are some shears like the ones with a swivel thumb or twister type handle that are very difficult to use without a ring in the thumb hole. Many times, your finger rings break or are missing. If you contact your sharpener, they usually have a selection of rings for you. The manufacturer of your shears would normally have some at their office they can send you.

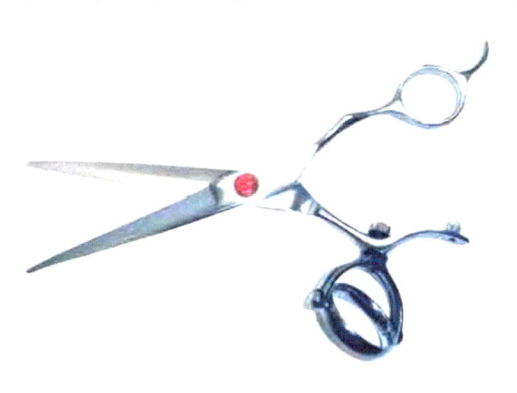

Shears like the Bonika Rocker with a swivel thumb is easier to maneuver with in insert ring in the thumb hole.

Grime and debris can get clogged under your rings and cause your shears to rust. Occasionally remove your ring carefully and clean it and the

> **DIY Idea** - If a plastic hard finger ring is too big and hard to fit in the shear, heating it with a hair dryer can soften it so that it will go in easier.

finger hole of your shears. A little oil between the ring and the shear will protect the shear and make it easier to slide the ring back into place.

A jelly gummy type ring can often be massaged and manipulated to fit. If it can't be massaged into position, a small section of the ring can be cut out using an Exacto™ knife or a razor blade. This works best on the thicker jelly type rings. I've seen modified rings like these last for years.

If an insert ring is too small to fit your shears, tape or a band-aid can be wrapped around the handle hole first then the insert ring put into place. A pretty ribbon will also work to make the hole smaller before inserting the finger ring.

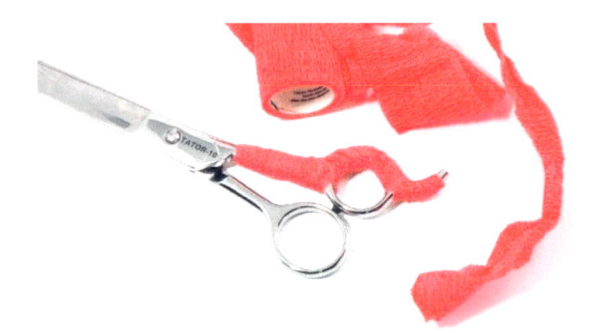

Self-adherent bandage wrapped around the finger hole and shank can customize the shear and provide extra grip.

> **DIY Idea** - If you don't have a ring, a self-adherent bandage roll found at any pharmacy works well. Wrap it around the rings and even the shanks of the shears. You can find these in assorted colors as well.

A few weeks ago, while visiting a salon here in Atlanta, I was given a shear to sharpen from one of the stylists who had traveled to Korea to take an advanced cutting. The instructor had taken her shears and applied a thin leather strap to wrap the shank and the finger hole. She had this on her shears for over a year. It was useful and distinctive. The leather had taken on an attractive rustic patina with age. To make this craft for your shears, purchase a roll of thin leather cord from a hobby store. You will need real leather for this instead of imitation leather. Wet the leather and stretch it while wrapping it around the shank, finger hole and even finger rest of the shears. Secure if needed with a touch of glue. Let it dry and shrink into place. This will give a secure grip to the shears while making the finger hole smaller. The feel of real leather is a rich texture to your hand giving a firm grip. If you tend to drop your shears this may be something you may want to try.

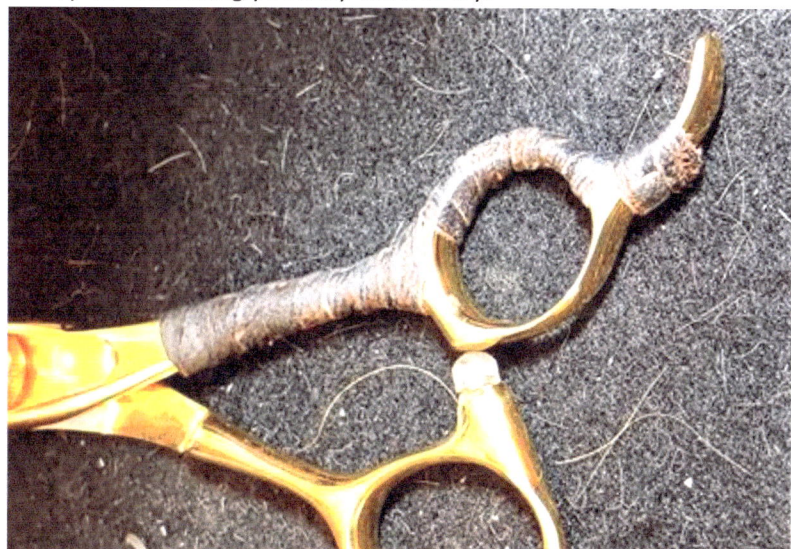

Leather wrap seen on a stylist shear.

11
HOW TO TELL IF YOUR SHEARS ARE DULL

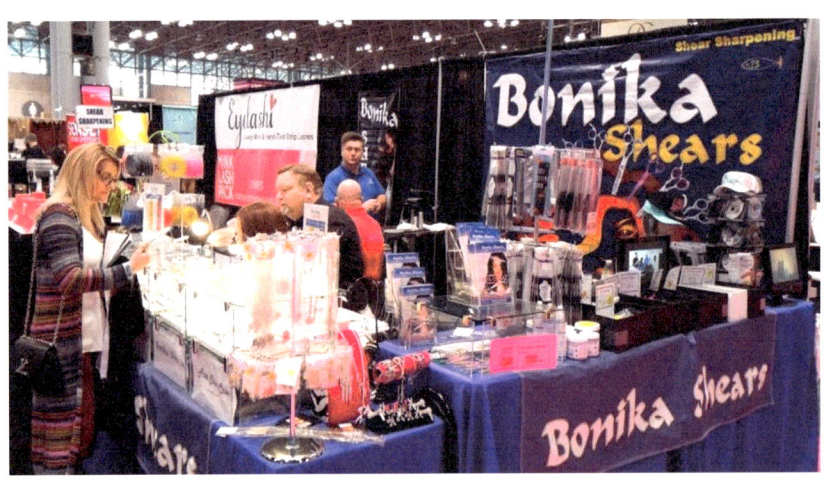

We were at the Premiere Orlando Hair Show a few years back and a stylist came to our booth and said, "I think it's time to replace my shears. I bought them from you eight years ago, but they are not cutting well."

My husband said, "That could be a warranty issue. When was the last time you had them sharpened?"

"Sharpened? I've never had them sharpened."

"Well," Gene said, "I think that might be your problem right there."

He could have told her she was not very sharp as well, but he is a lot more tactful than I. Anytime your shears are not cutting well and it has been a few months since they were serviced or purchased, your edges may have dulled.

There was another incident where I sold a new pair of shears to a stylist in a new shop near my home. She called me two weeks later claiming her new shears were already dull. I went by and sure enough, there were nicks all down the blade. Curious, I asked her, "How much cutting *have* you been doing?"

She said, "I've been pretty busy. Do you see all the new buildings going in across the street? All those guys have been coming in for a haircut."

"Did you cut their hair dry? Did you wash their hair first?"

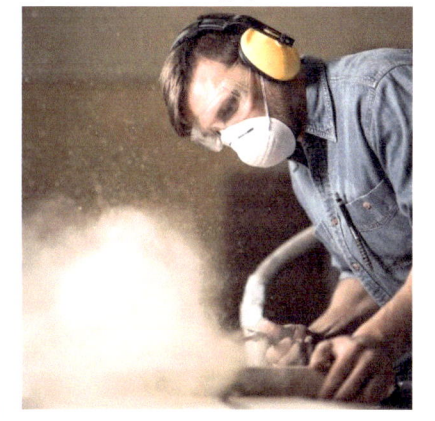

"No, they were in a hurry."

"Was there dry-wall and saw dust in their hair?" I asked.

"Well, ….. maybe….,"

Shears are made to cut hair, not sawdust, beach sand or other things that might be hanging around on the scalp.

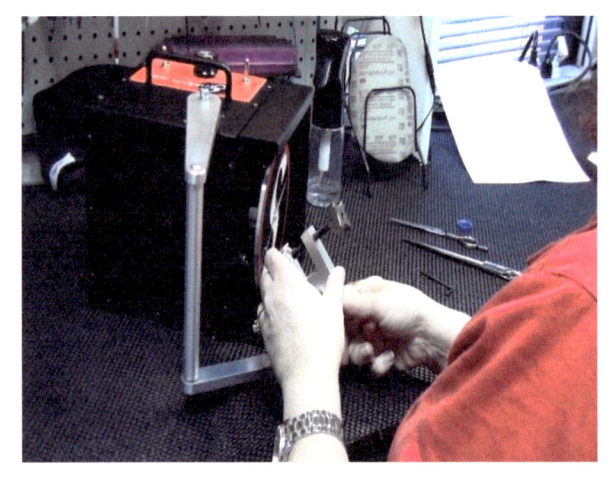

Have your shears sharpened when they need it. That is usually less than four years and it could be in two weeks. Typically, stylists will call the sharpener when the shears they are using are too dull to cut properly. It's best to be proactive and not reactive when it comes to sharpening.

If you wait too long these things can occur:

You must work your hands harder to cut the hair.

The hair will chew or pull causing damage to the hair resulting in split ends.

The sharpener may not be available causing you to wait even longer for sharpening.

The cuts can be uneven if the shears tend to fold before they cut.

You will be more likely to cut yourself because you chase the hair.

Cuts with dull shears hurt more and heal more slowly than cuts with sharp shears.

Long before these problems set in, you should check your shears periodically to see if the edge has dulled. Depending on the shears brand and metal quality it would be good to check your sharpness every two weeks after the first three months.

Test for Sharpness

How should you objectively test your shears to see if you need to have them sharpened? As you know you should never use your good stylist shears to cut paper. However, it will not harm your edges if you create special testing paper by separating out an inexpensive (not the extra strong lotion type) Puff™ Tissue to a single ply. Cut the tissue with your shears (using light pressure – no side pressure) and see if you get a clean cut all the way to the tip. If they do not cut, double check the adjustment and try again.

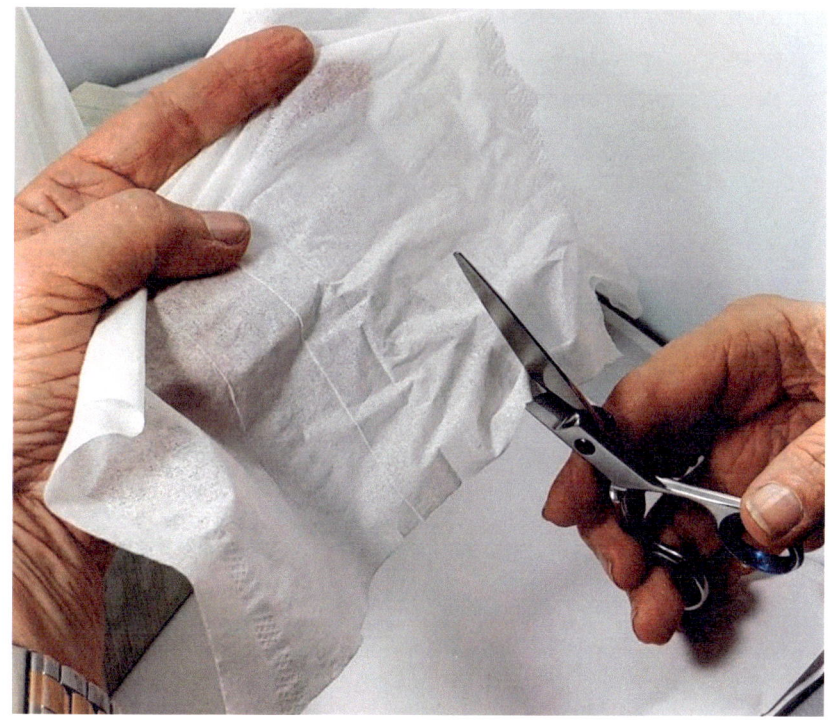

Cut single ply Puff™ tissue to see if your shears need sharpening.

There is additional testing needed if you use your shears for slide cutting and need very sharp shears. Do the same tissue test on dampened tissue. Spray the tissue using your water bottle and cut the dampened tissue slowly using the least pressure possible. If the paper tears instead of cuts, there are nicks in the blade and it's time to call the sharpener.

💡 *DIY Idea – Before you have your shears professionally sharpened you may be able to restore the edge with a nail buffer. Fine nail buffers are 3000 grit. Do not get an emery board this is too rough. With the shears open, use light pressure and stroke the blades of your shears toward the edge following the curve of the outside blade. Repeat on the inside sliding the buffer flat in a diagonal motion from the pivot to the tip moving toward the sharp edge. Repeat this twice and check the cut. If it has improved but does not cut cleanly, try the process again. If it still does not cut to the tip*

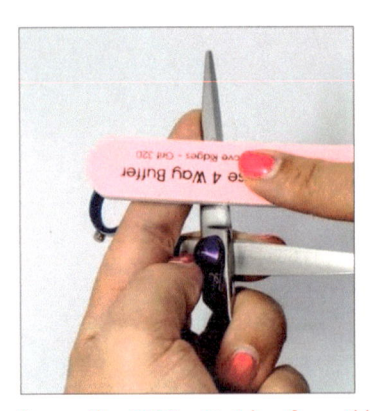

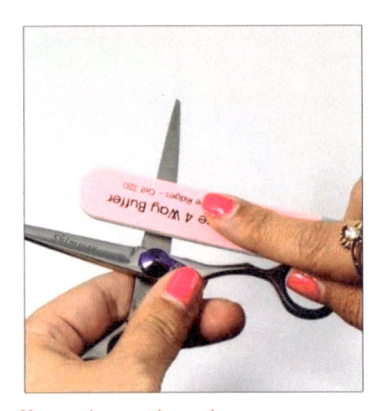

Gently use the 3000 grit side of a nail buffer to hone the edge.

Anytime your shears will not perform correctly, it is time to call the professional sharpener. Keep in mind that sharpening will shorten the life of your shears. Each time they are sharpened, metal is removed so that it will reach the point that your shears need to be retired. It is not good to postpone sharpening when your shears need it, but it is unwise to over sharpen your shears as well.

Some shear manufacturers and sharpeners sell contracts to have shears sharpened on a regular basis. These contracts can be useful since they allow the stylist to budget and both the sharpener and the stylist have a regular schedule. However, if the sharpeners and companies selling these contracts have little training, they will remove too much metal and shorten the life of your shears.

> *DIY Idea –No Puff™ tissue? Although it is not as good you can alternately use Kleenex or single ply toilet paper. This is a case where the lower the quality, the thinner the tissue, the better it is for a sharpening test.*

Most of the time the stylist will not save money using the contracts since they will often have their shears sharpened more often than is necessary. Even the companies that advertise they sharpen without abrasives or with lasers will remove metal. Sharpening requires metal removal to take out nicks, create a bur and bring up an edge. Even very fine grit sharpening is using an abrasive. Don't be fooled by salesmen who sell sharpening contracts without an understanding of the sharpening process.

How do You Know if Your Shears are Too Old or Too Worn Out to Sharpen?

The main indication that your shears are beyond repair is when the blade has been sharpened away to the point where the edges will not meet properly. This will usually happen when $1/4^{th}$ to $1/3^{rd}$ of the blade is removed. The rideline which is the shiny edge along the inside of the cutting blade is now appearing on the back side of the blade instead of the edge.

When these signs appear, it may be time to retire your shears. This will most likely occur after 4 to 10 years of use depending on the sharpening, care and quality of the shears. One bad sharpening can remove so much metal that they are beyond repair after one sharpening. A quality shear that is taken care of without a history of dropping and nicks and sharpened by a well-equipped and trained sharpener can go beyond 20 years performing well.

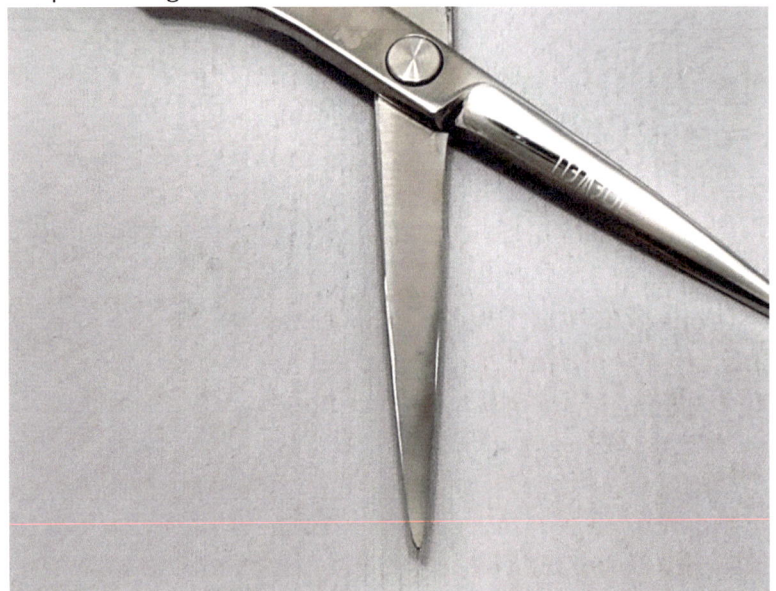

This shear has been over sharpened and sharpened incorrectly. It might not be repairable. Notice the rideline on the backside of the blade.

DIY Idea – Over sharpened shears with tips that don't meet can sometimes be corrected by trimming the bumper. Use a nail nipper or razor blade to trim off a little of the rubber. You can also use a lighter to heat the rubber bumper then squeeze the handle closed to where the tips meet and let the bumper cool. This will only work if you have enough rubber on your bumper.

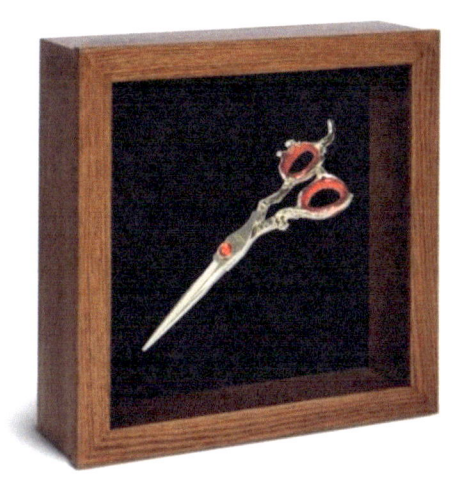

If your shears are at the retirement age and you are unwilling to part with them, master trained sharpeners can repair these shears by realigning or chaffering the pivot area. This is advanced mechanical work and involves a risk of breaking the shears.

The best idea is to buy a pretty shadow box. Put your prize shears in the box and hang them on the wall so you can reminisce about the joy, the beautiful haircuts and all the money those shears brought to you. Then go out and bless yourself with a new pair.

DIY Idea – If you are a stylist who gets overly attached to one particular shear, buy some back-ups of the same make and model. If you shear is already a discontinued shear, check out some of the resale sites or post inquiries on stylists chat boards. Roberta Marshall, top educator for Bronner Brothers Professional has 3 pairs of the Bonika Firefly shears because she loves it so much.

12

HOW TO FIND A SHARPENER

A good local sharpener can be as much an asset to your shears as a good car mechanic is to your car. You need someone who is available. Someone you can trust. Someone who knows how to care for your favorite shears.

Surprisingly enough sending your shears back to the manufacturer is not always the best solution. There are many sharpeners throughout the United States and urban areas throughout the world. Many mobile and local sharpeners are well equipped and trained and can give you customized sharpening right in your salon better than the manufacturer can supply. They know how you cut and how you hold your shears. They learn what you expect your shears to do for you and can often customize the edge to suit your needs. This edge may not be exactly what the factory put on your shears if you are using your shears in a unique method.

There are other sharpeners who are poorly trained, poorly equipped and even dishonest and frankly, creepy. You want to avoid these sharpeners and not even have them into your shop! How do you find the sharpener that is best for your shears?

There are stories I know to be true of sharpeners. I know one sharpener who told me he was offended by some remark by the stylist. He said he deliberately wrecked a pair of shears with one of his coarse files and walked out.

There was another man, here in the Atlanta area who was a drug addict. He would convince stylists he could sharpen shears and pretended to be working for us. He would take the shears out and scrape them on the sidewalk. The stylist would pay without checking them first and he walked out with their money.

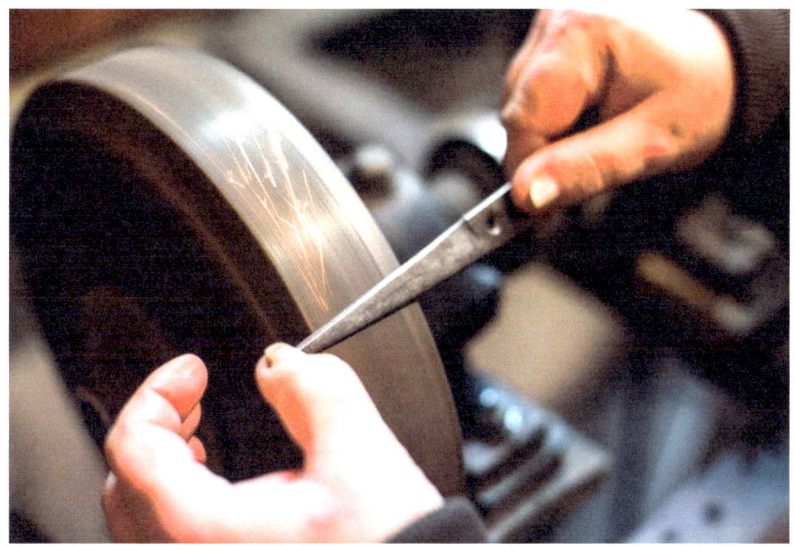

This shear will be ruined if sharpened like this. Be sure your sharpener is professionally trained and equipped.

Another horror story was about a woman here in the Atlanta area who bought a knife sharpener online and went around sharpening beauty shears on a knife sharpener. This really damaged some shears.

Many salons in resort areas near interstates can expect roaming sharpeners to stop in from other areas of the country. They can claim all kinds of expertise and they may be very good. They may also have just purchased a $800 grinding type sharpener and watched a one hour video and are now practicing on your precious tools. So, what steps should you take in looking for a sharpener for your shears?

Look for a Specialist

Stylist shears are the most delicate and sophisticated of tools that need sharpening. Sharpeners who sharpen a variety of tools like ice skates, meat cleavers, drill bits, and lawnmower blades rarely have the time to specialize in beauty shears. Usually a sharpener who specializes in sharpening shears and scissors are better than general sharpers. The sharpeners who specialize in beauty industry shears rather than groomers scissors and clipper blades are in most cases better as well.

Check Online

Research on the internet for sharpeners in your area. Look for certifications and registrations. Websites of sharpeners often show their credentials, training and photos of their equipment. Go to sharpener look-ups like www.findasharpener.com or websites of sharpening organizations to find a sharpener. Ask in stylist groups on Facebook if they recommend a sharpener.

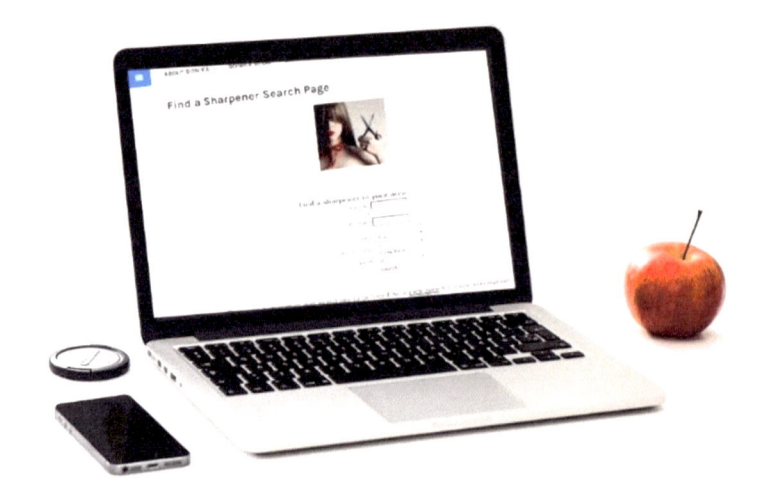

Check with Other Stylists

Ask for recommendations from the stylists in your salon and stylists in salons near you. The local beauty supply store may have cards of sharpeners you can check out.

When looking for recommendations from stylists ask the individuals who have very expensive shears and are picky as to their care of their tools. Some stylists may be perfectly satisfied with a sharpener which would not be of the quality that another stylist would demand.

Give them a Test Shear

Give the sharpener a test shear first before they get your expensive shears. See if their sharpening was able to make the shears cut again.

When we were at the Premiere Orlando Hair show earlier this year, four stylists from Georgia brought their shears to our booth for sharpening. Each stylist had 3 to 4 shears. All had been sharpened incorrectly with the convex edge changed to a bevel and the rideline removed. My sharpener, Jay Hunter, was able to successfully restore them, but he was not able to add metal back. The life expectancy of all these shears were drastically decreased. If they had given this new sharpener one shear to sharpen then checked it and cut with it a few weeks before giving them all the shears for the salon, they would have saved themselves a lot of problems. Never give a new sharpener all your shears. Test them out first before you can completely trust them.

Look at the Equipment

A professional shear sharpener should have professional expensive looking equipment. It should be dusty. If it is pristine, they may be new to sharpening.

Beauty shear sharpeners should be using a belt sander or flathone system since this is what they use in the factories of Japan and other Asian countries making quality beauty shears. Mobile sharpeners will most likely have a flathone system since the belt-sander that is large enough for shears will be too bulky, dusty and noisy to bring into a salon. The traditional grinder type equipment as seen in the local hardware store is used by many mobile sharpeners. This may be sufficient if you have a bevel edge shear. If you have a Japanese type shear with a convex edge this equipment will change the shape of the edge. There are new designs of shear sharpening equipment that are being introduced to the market. I will refrain from passing judgement except to say I prefer to sharpen in a way most closely the same as the way shears are originally sharpened in the manufacturing process.

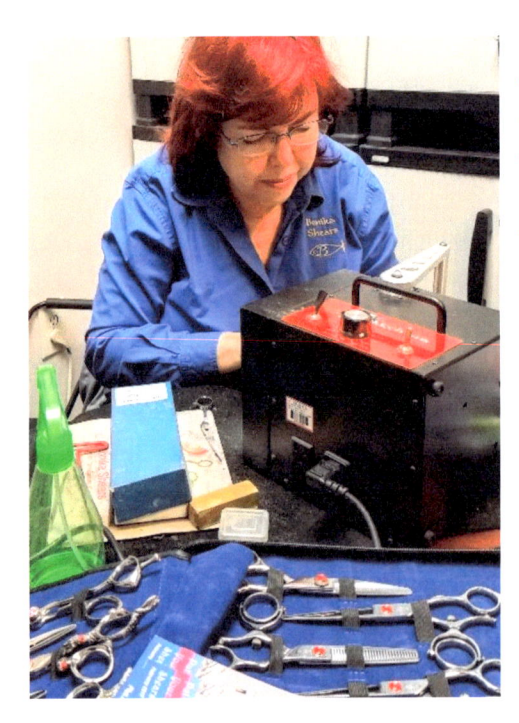

The author sharpening inside a salon using the Scimech™ Flathone System. Notice the shears set out on the table. The most successful sharpeners sell shears while they are sharpening.

Our company markets and recommends the Scimech HD Scissor Flathone. This is not the only flathone system that will give an excellent edge. Just like in hair cutting, the shears are just a tool in the hands of a skilled and educated stylist. We also recommend that beauty shears be sharpened using a clamp or jig device that will maintain a consistent and precise angle. Wet or dampened abrasive plates is desirable since it will keep the blades from overheating which can affect the temper or hardness of the steel. The inside edge should be honed by hand on a separate waterstone of smooth abrasive instead of using mechanical equipment. Once again there are new devices and machinery always being designed that are different than the manufacturing in Japan. Anything very different than the factory methods should be fully vetted before you allow them to sharpen your shears.

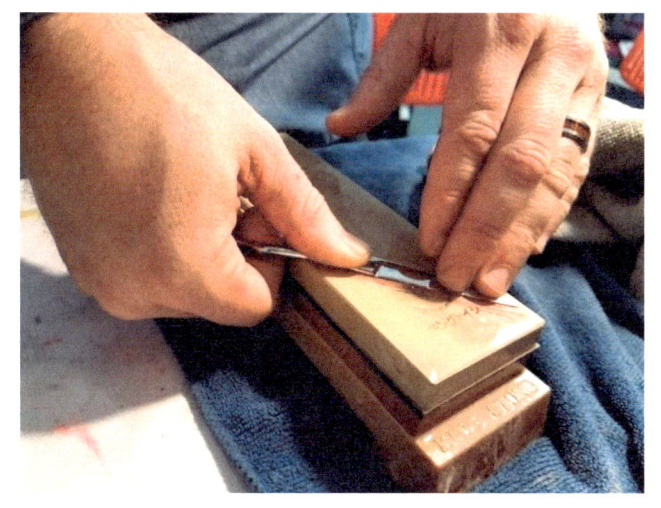

Inside of a shear is being hand honed on a high grit, very smooth Japanese Waterstone.

Where was the sharpener trained?

Sharpening training can come in a variety of methods from YouTube to scissor production factories. It is hard to know whether a sharpener has been properly trained, however, most who have gone through a formal training will typically have a certificate of some kind. The best training is on-going training. Just like in the hair industry the real knowledge of hair cutting comes from experience, practice and advanced classes. Sharpeners who care about their craft will have some basic initial training as well as advanced classes from sharpening conventions and private classes.

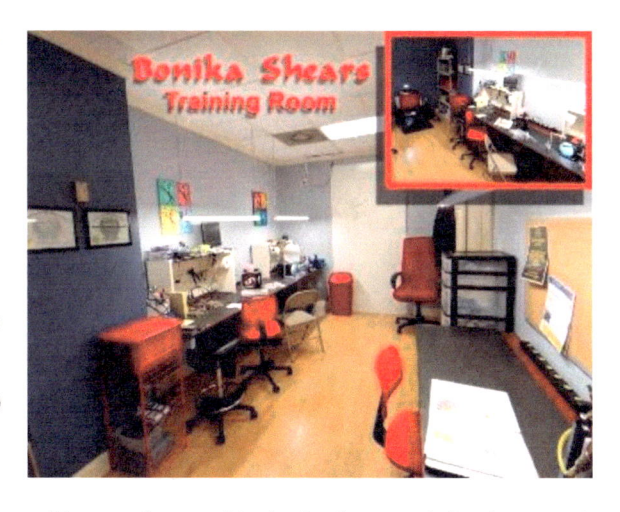

Interview your sharpener and ask about their equipment and training as well as experience.

> **DIY Idea – Get this information yourself. Stalk your potential new sharpener on Facebook and Instagram. The information will generally be available for inspection on the website or Facebook page of the local sharpener you are considering.**

What to do if you can't find a decent sharpener in your area?

If you have used all diligence and can't find a mobile sharpener that meets your approval, don't risk your expensive shears with a subpar sharpener. You might want to use them for your back-up shears or older shears, but your better shears should be sent out. Find out what sharpener your brand of shears recommends. This would be your first choice. You can also inquire in stylist chat rooms on social media to get recommendations.

There are times when you should have your shears sharpened by mail-order rather than use a local sharpener. Just because a sharpener accepts mail-order sharpening does not mean they will do a great job on your shears. Even mail-order sharpeners should be fully vetted as well. Our company accepts mail-order sharpening and will email you a prepaid shipping label. Get your label at http://bonika.com/sharpening. There are many other reputable mail-order sharpening locations as well.

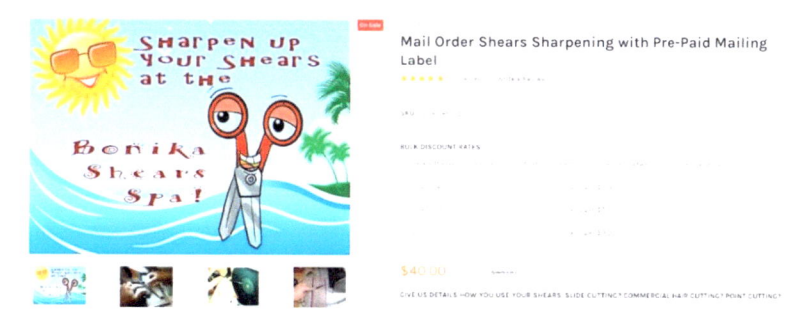

When you ship your shears, it is important that you send them correctly. First be sure the shears will not open in shipping. Wrap them in bubble wrap. Do not use tape on the shears themselves as this is hard to clean off and can trap moisture to the edge causing corrosion. Once wrapped put them in a box. A USPS small Priority mailbox is free from your post office and gives good protection to your shears. Refer to chapter eight on how to pack your shears.

Before you seal the box, put in your payment (not cash) your name, address, phone number and email address. Also include other helpful instruction.

Typical helpful instruction might be:

- Be sure the tips are rounded ... or be sure the tips are pointy.
- I need one blade serrated, please.
- I like to slide cut ... or I like to point cut.
- Please replace the insert sizer rings.
- Please replace the finger rest …. Or don't replace the finger rest.
- Please glue on the finger rest, it keeps coming loose.
- These scissors are old, they were my mother's. Please shine them up, I plan to put them in a shadow box.

Become a Professional Shear Sharpener Yourself

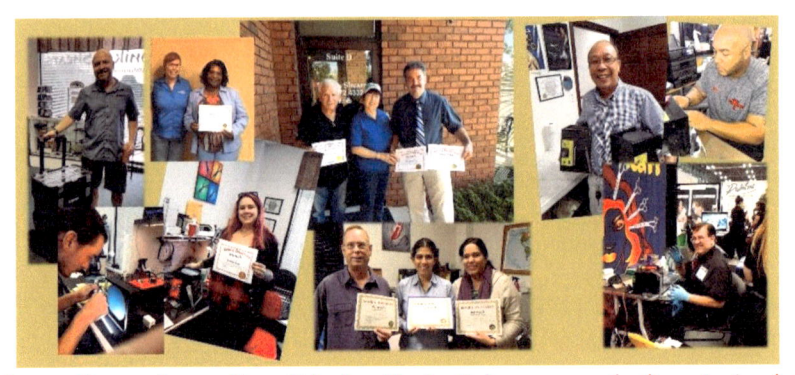

Photos of a small sampling of the hundreds of sharpeners who have trained at our Bonika Shears training facility. If you want more information on becoming a professional sharpener contact the author or go to www.bonika.com.

 The ultimate DIY idea is to become a shear sharpener yourself. How many beauty shops are in your area? Did you know that beauty shear sharpeners can earn a serious income? Stylist pay immediately $25 to $30 per shear. They have an average of 4 shears sharpened two to three times per year and buy more shears from their sharpeners. This is a one person business with little or no overhead and very low start-up cost. You can set-up inside the beauty salons with no need to buy a van.

A small investment can set you on a fun, lucrative and challenging path. If this is not a direction for your gifts and talents you might suggest this to someone else in your life. In our training facilities sharpeners come of all ages and backgrounds, although most are spouses, friends or siblings of stylists. Get your training from the same company that sells you the equipment. Look for a company that will supplement your training with ongoing seminars, training manuals, videos and easy phone access for questions when you are in the field.

13

SPECIALTY SHEARS DIY TIPS

Left-Handed Shears

Left-handed stylists should be using left-handed shears to prolong the health of their hand. Many left-handed stylists like beauty educator **Dave Ray** of Beauty Werkz have taught themselves to use both left and right-handed shears. Many of the specialty shears are only available in a right-handed version. Left-handed people are limited in their creativity if they can only use left-handed shears. However, choosing the shear they use for the majority of their haircutting, these should be of the left-handed variety.

True left-handed shears will cross backwards. Some manufacturers produce left-handed shears which are right-handed shears with the screw designed so that the adjustable thumb-nut screw head can be put on either side for the convenience of the left-handed stylist. It is important that you recognize a left-handed shear even if you are not left-handed. There have been several times that I have met right-handed stylists that were sold or given left-handed shears and wondered why they were unable to cut hair.

Dave Ray on stage at the Premiere Orlando Hair Show using a righthanded pair of curved shears in his left hand.

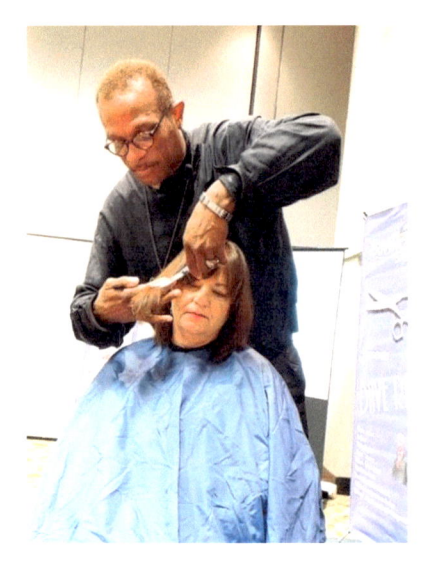

A true left-handed shear will have the sharp edge of the blade on top on the left side. This will be true even if the blades are turned over. If the shears are facing you with the tips up and the handles next to your body, the blade on top, facing you will cross the bottom blade diagonally from the left to the right. A right-handed shear will be the opposite.

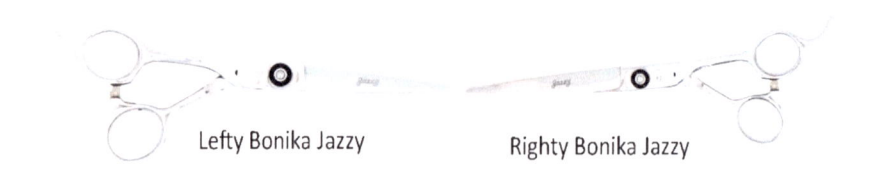

Lefty Bonika Jazzy   Righty Bonika Jazzy

Left-handed shears must be sharpened in a different way. Sharpeners must work the shears from a different direction. This is hard to do if the sharpener is a "free-hand" sharpener and doesn't have a jig or clamping system that will adapt to a lefty shear. In addition, sharpeners must hold them in their left hand to test them.

Zoe Lambert wrote on the Facebook chat Stylist 911 with **Mags Kavanaugh** "I take my shears to get sharpened by a left-handed shear sharpener. It's much harder for right-handed sharpeners to test if my shears work the right way." This may not always be necessary, but it is true a left-handed sharpener would have a better understanding and feel for making her shears cut best for her left hand. **Don Jun**, a Korean shear expert said when he was manufacturing shears, he never produced any left-handed shears in his factory because he didn't have any left-handed sharpeners in his plant.

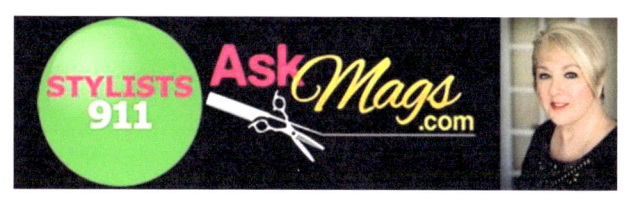

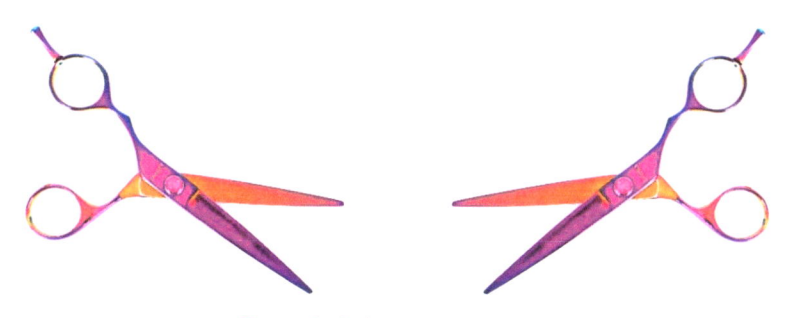

Left-Handed Shears are on the left.

Left-handed stylists must always cut with shears before they purchase. The variants between the hand finishing of shears is augmented for left-handed shears. I would never recommend buying shears without trying them first, especially for a left-handed person.

DIY Idea – Sometimes left-handed shears perform better when the pivot screw is adjusted a little tighter.

Curved Shears

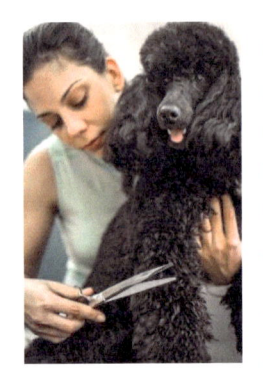

Curved shears have been used for years by groomers and urban barbers. In the late 90's curved shears brought over from the groomers to the beauty industry became very popular. Since then, there has been improvements made to the curved shears used by stylists.

The benefits of using curved shears is many. Curved shears follow the curve of the head or can go opposite to the head shape to achieve different effects. They also aid in point cutting and cutting curly hair. Emmy nominated stylist, **Yancey Edwards** of Shear Insanity Salon in New Jersey was one of the first people to begin using the curved shears when making deep textured cuts into weave and commercial hair. He likes the longer blades where some stylists are more comfortable with a shorter shear.

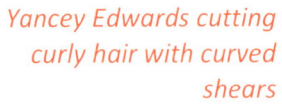

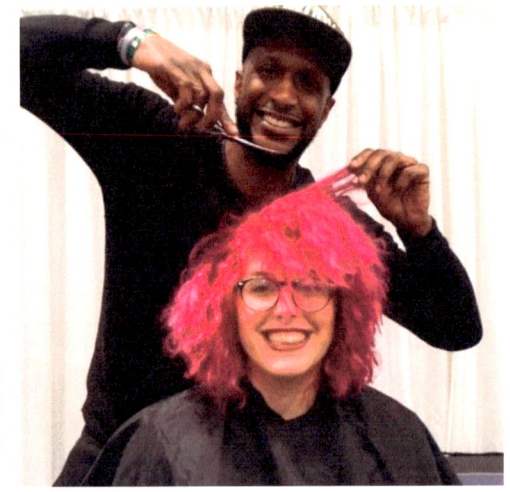

Yancey Edwards cutting curly hair with curved shears

Most people, including sharpeners, do not realize curved blade shears are made straight in the factory. After they are finished and sharpened, the curve is put in mechanically into the shears. This means that it is impossible to resharpen a curve shear in the exact way it was made. Curved shears are one of the most difficult types of shears for sharpening. They typically will need replacing more often than other shears.

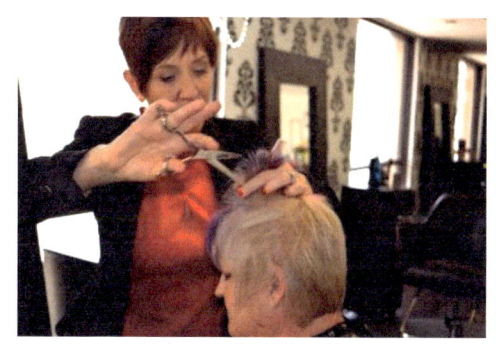

Stylist Robin DeMarchi of West Virginia cutting texture into hair with her curved shears.

Very often a curved shear will have a drag area where they close easily then the blades appear to rub and feel tight. This is a common occurrence and usually is in the area where the blade arcs. The bad news is the only way to fix this is to bend the blade, so the alignment or set is corrected. The good news is that these shears are almost impossible to break when resetting the alignment because they were designed to be bent in the original manufacturing process. I don't recommend that someone untrained should try realigning curved shears.

It is better to prevent this misalignment condition from occurring than fixing it afterwards. Don't cut large chunks of hair with your curved shears. This can push the blades too far apart affecting the alignment. Also don't have the curved shears in a soft case and place something heavy on them. This flattens the curve of the blades and creates the problem.

How do you know whether you have bought beauty industry curved shears or ones designed for the grooming industry? Usually, groomer curved shears used on poodles and other breeds of dogs will have a blunter edge and will curve down in the direction away from the face of the shear. Stylist curved shears typically will curve up toward the top of the shear although there are exceptions.

Stylist curved shears typically curve up

Barbers like curved shears because they can follow the shape of the head. Stylists like to point cut and sculpt the hair using their curved shears in a variety of ways. The stylist's curved shears will often have a sharper edge, sometimes convex, creating a smoother, quieter cutting action.

Groomer / barber style curved shear.

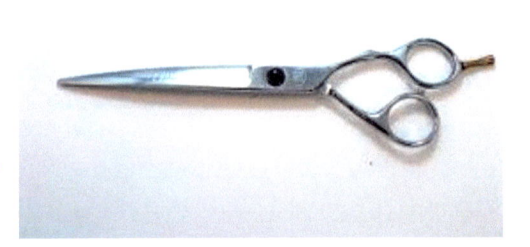

Texturizers and Thinners

All stylists and barbers are issued a pair of thinning shears when they are in school. These shears are not used as often and will be used in different ways for different results. The terminology for thinning shears will vary. How do you know the difference between a thinning shear, a blending shear and a texturizing shear?

In the manufacturing end of the business a thinning shear or *thinner* technically is one with teeth on both sides.

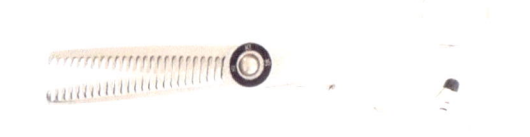

Thinning Shear

A blending shear or *blender* is a shear with fine teeth on one side.

Blending Shear

A texturizing shear or *texturizer* is a blending shear with fewer teeth, usually 5 - 20 teeth. The texturizers with large chunky teeth, usually five teeth are often called channeling shears or *channelers*. Occasionally they are referred to as *chunkers*.

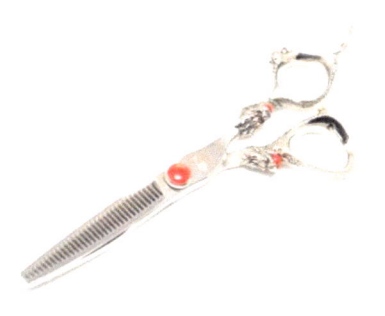

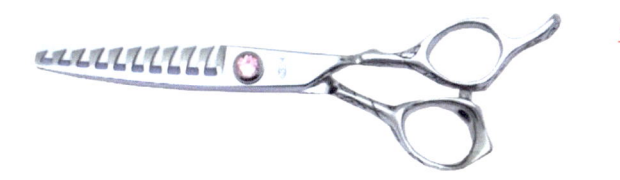

10 tooth texturizer

From a stylist point of view, any or all, of these types of shears can be used for any of these three purposes. Hair that is cut near the scalp, just beyond the "bend line" will thin the hair. It removes bulk and heaviness. (the *bend line* is where the hair bends, cutting closer to the scalp will make it stand up... unless of course that is what you want to accomplish).

Texture cutting is in the center of the shaft of hair, it is placed in specific locations to achieve various looks from spikes to froth to wispys. Blending is at the ends of the hair to create invisible layers, so the hair appears to be one length. Blending with a texture shear can remove the weight line in a men's cut after clippering creating a polished yet textured affect.

So, whether you call your tools blenders, thinners or texturizers, all these shears have teeth. Shears with teeth or a comb will normally require less

> **DIY Idea** – Often fine-toothed blending shears will have debris accumulate between the teeth. Keep a toothbrush handy and give your shears teeth a good brushing.

care than other shears for the simple reason they are used less and tend to have a blunter, stronger edge. There are, however, problems that are unique to these shears that can be dealt with effectively.

What to do if your shears pull hair when cutting. If your shears are pulling hair this could be due to a number of reasons. The most common is that the shears are dull. Before calling the sharpener, try the nail buffer technique as described in chapter twelve. If they click when you close them, see if the bumper is gone. A missing bumper can cause the blades to close so that the hair is pinched between the two blades. Replace the bumper (see chapter ten) and check how your shears cut now. If they are still pulling hair, call your sharpener. Shears that pull hair can cause you to lose a client.

What to do if your shears won't close. If your shears don't close or the tooth bites into the other blade you may have a bent tooth. A bent tooth can be carefully straightened using needle nose pliers. If the tooth breaks off, the shears are still useable. They won't cut in that section but the rest of the shears will cut well. This is some extreme DIY care on your shears and might be better left to a professional.

There was a popular technique a few years ago of pulling all the hair up into a ponytail, twisting the ponytail, then cutting into the twist with your texturizer shears. This looked good on stage by the platform artist. However, the abuse to the shears would create a problem where the teeth would hang up and the shears would not close properly. Because of the thin nature of the blades this was a problem that could sometimes be honed away by a sharpener but more often than not was not fixable.

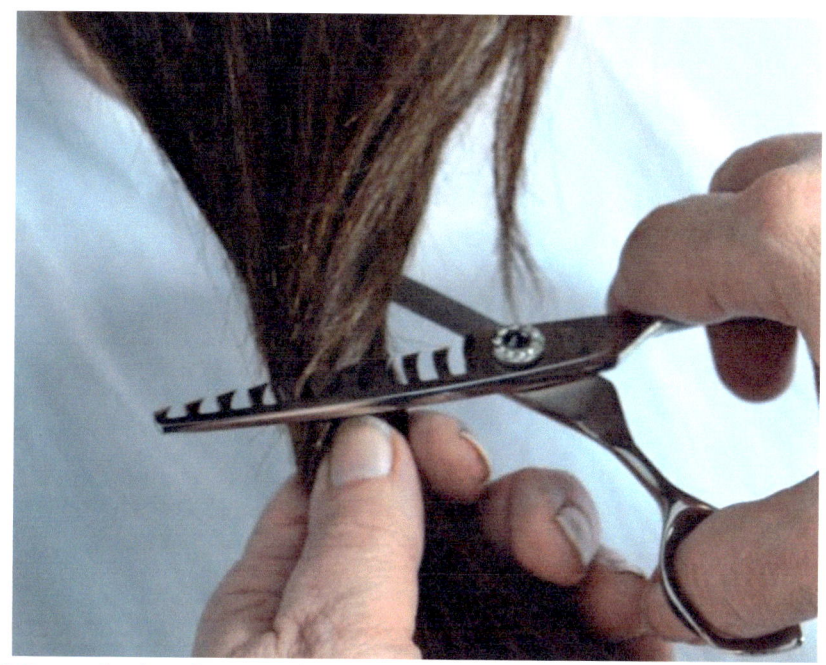

Point cutting into the twisted hair ends with a texturizer, curve or other shears will not harm the shears. Cutting into the twisted compressed hair as pictured can cause great damage to the alignment of the blades and the handle.

What to do if your shears are bending hair. If your thinners or blenders are making the hair bend or flip rather than cutting there is one of two things most likely happening. The easiest problem to fix is to check the adjustment of the screw. Tighten the screw a small amount and see if this helps. If it improves without fixing the problem, tighten it some more. This is usually the culprit for thinners that bend hair.

If the screw adjustment did not fix the shears your blades are not coming together correctly. This is typically an alignment problem and should be handled by a professional sharpener. This is not always repairable and

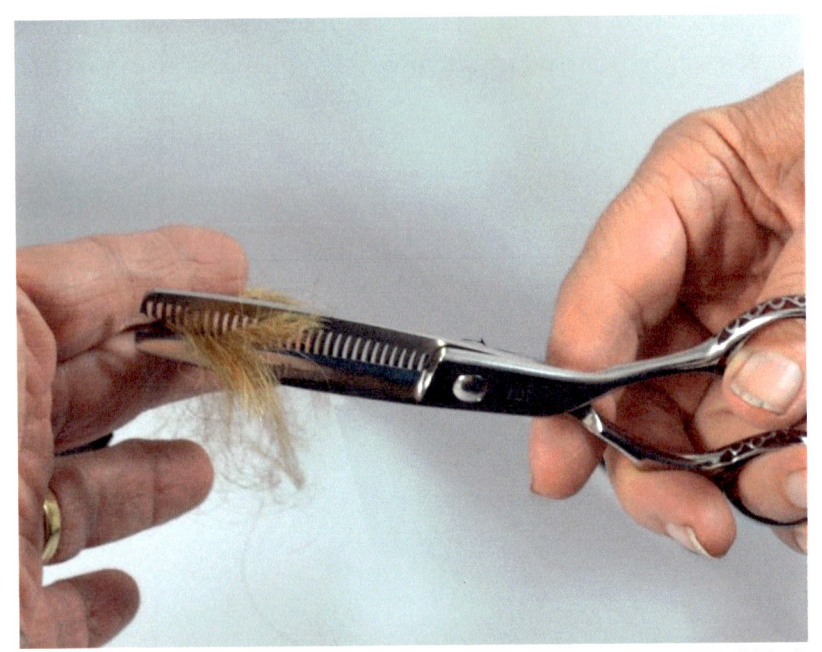

Notice how the hair flips or bends. This can be either a loose screw, dull blade or a misalignment of the blades. Tighten the screw to see if this corrects the problem.

most likely was caused by dropping the shears or cutting larger chunks of hair than the shears were intended to cut.

14
CONCLUSION

I have come to be very philosophical about stylist shears. They are so much more than two knife blades held together by a screw. The mechanics and nuances continue to fascinate me after three decades of sharpening. The love affair between a stylist and their shears still fills me with wonder. My nearly fifty years of marriage I compare to a pair of shears. Two opposite but complementary individuals held together by God, working together as a team and cutting anything that comes between us. I think about shears. I paint pictures of shears. I wear earrings and bracelets that look like shears.

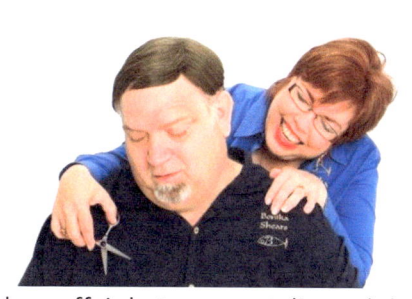

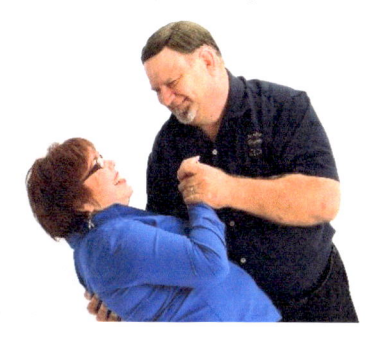

The author, Bonnie Megowan and her husband Gene Megowan

The tattoo on the back of this stylist was a copy of her favorite shear the Bonika Tribal designed by Jay Hunter.

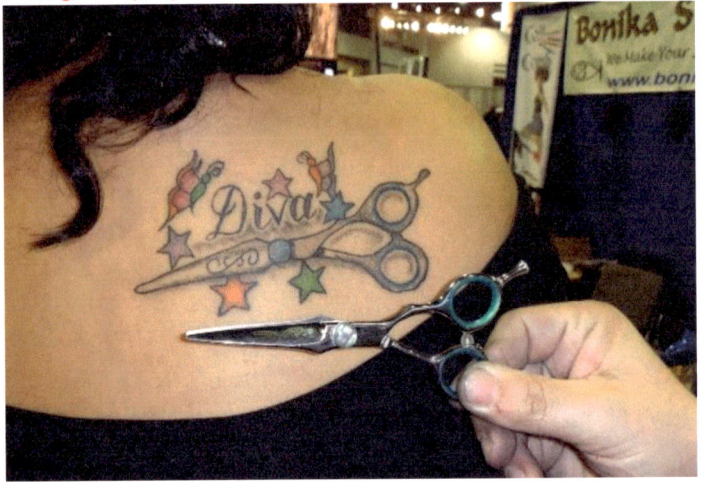

I am obsessed with collecting photos of stylist's tattoos where they paint the tool of their artistry permanently on their bodies. It is humbling and honoring when I find a shear the stylist has bought from me that they love so much they want to look at it forever. I have hundreds of these photos taken at various hairshows posted on the internet at facebook.com/scissortattoo.

Respect and care for your shears and they will respect and care for you. A little extra care and time spent with your shears will be time well invested.

What can a well performing shear do for you and your career and income?

Derek J, famous celebrity stylist here in Atlanta, is an example of how much a shear is worth. Derek has been on *Real Atlanta Housewives, Fashion Queens, Hair Battle Spectacular* and *Good Hair*. But before he became famous, he bought a $198.00 shear at our booth at a hair show. He entered the cutting contests at the show and won all three big money prize contests. That launched his career.

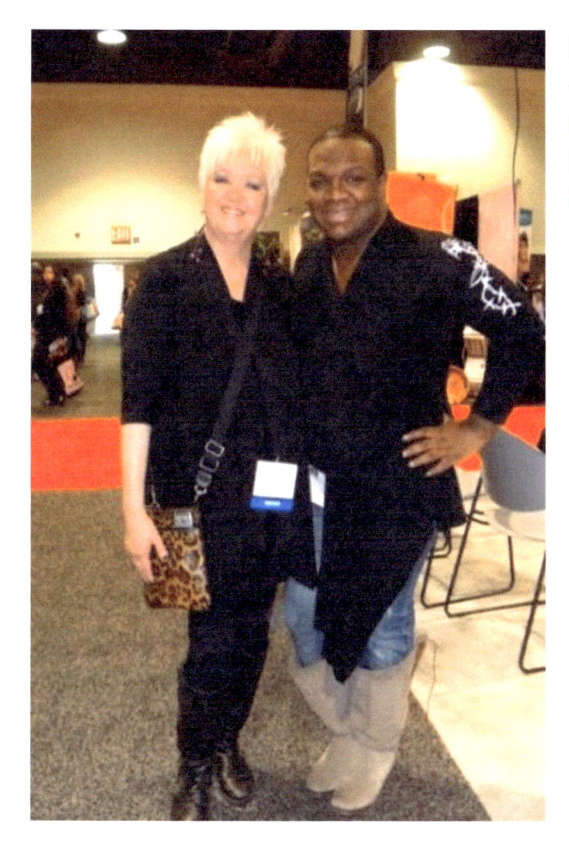

Derek J and Frances Dubois – both high income gorilla cutters pictured here at the International Beauty Show New York in 2012.

Derek is a gorilla cutter. His shears are always getting lost or stolen so he no longer has that original shear. But if he had kept it, and cared for it for the last fifteen years, that shear would have brought back a fortune. His base price for a haircut is $100 with everything a la carte. The price for a haircut increases with every additional shear or tool he picks up.

Let's break this down for the average stylist. If they bought a $198.00 shear like Derek and had it sharpened twice per year and kept it for ten years, that shear would cost a total of $798.00. If the stylist cuts 8 heads per day, 5 days per week, 50 weeks per year for 10 years, that is 20,000 haircuts. This would mean that shear would cost them only 4 cents per haircut.

According to the Professional Beauty Association the cost of average haircut in the USA in 2019 is $43.00. If that stylist was charging $43.00 per haircut, that shear would have earned that stylist $860,000.00 in those ten years.

Respect, love and be good to your shears. They are your money making machine and they work hard for you.

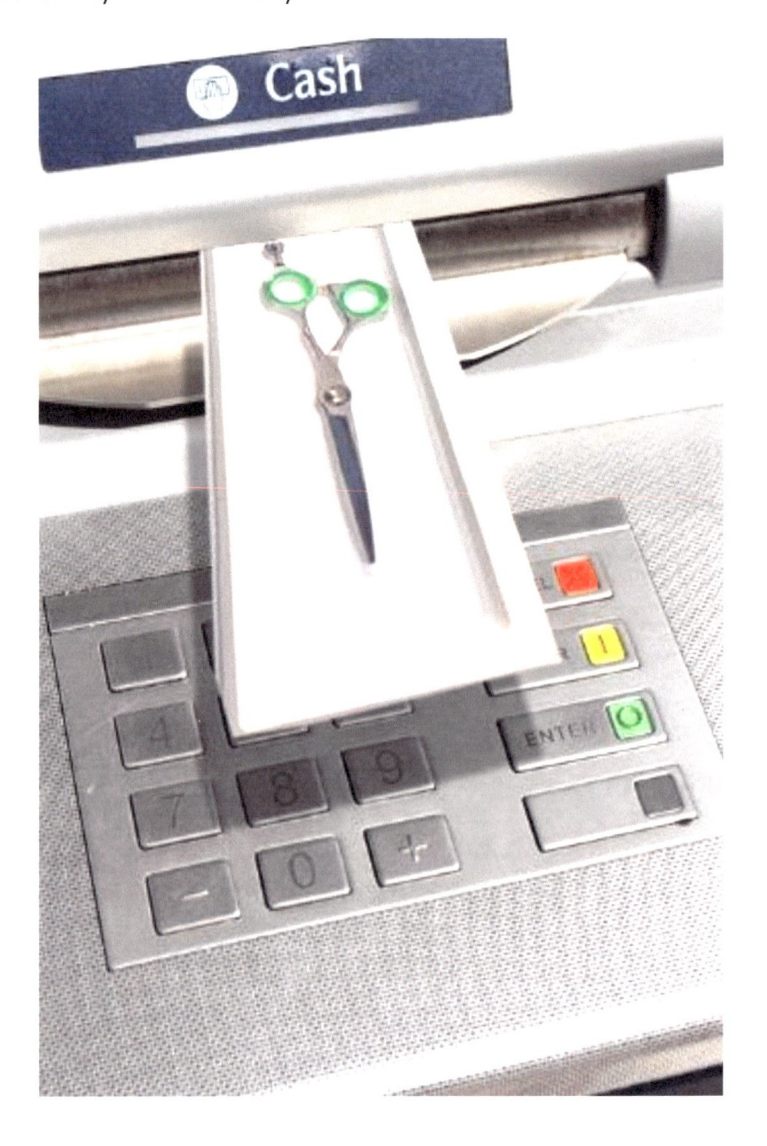

ABOUT THE AUTHOR

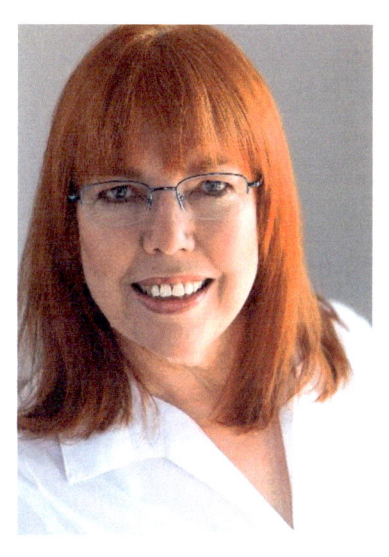

Bonnie Megowan is the CEO of Bonika Shears which is one of the premiere shear companies in the USA. She did not start as a sharpener or a stylist. Bonnie began her career as a high school science teacher. She continues to teach, not science, but in her new arena of shear sharpening, For the last 30 plus years she has sharpened shears in hair salons in the Atlanta, GA area. She has also become proficient in clipper blade sharpening as well. However, her true love is still teaching. She has taught sharpening to hundreds of men and women of all ages. They come from around the world to her private sharpening classes and group classes. In addition to teaching sharpening, she and her husband Gene lecture at various sharpening conventions and cosmetology schools. She writes articles for both stylist and sharpening publications.

The practical DIY know how has come from both experience and sharing with other sharpeners and stylists who have created hacks for overcoming a lack of tools or parts. Many times, as a mobile sharpener, she had to improvise when she didn't have a certain tool or part.

She was forced to do the most improvising in 1996. This was the year that Atlanta hosted the Olympic Games. Bonnie was involved in the recruitment of the stylists and barbers that worked in the Olympic hair salon in the Olympic Village. As a benefit she was able to work as the receptionist / tool repair person in the salon. Athletes had the ability to

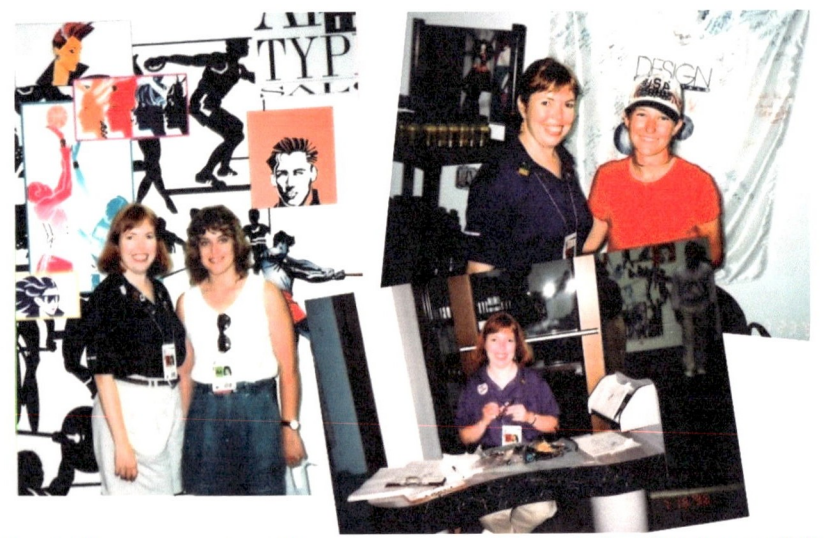

Bonnie Megowan posing with medal winning athletes at the All Hair types Salon in the Olympic Village. Bonnie sitting at the reception desk sharpening shears by hand.

use the salon for shampoos and haircuts as often as they liked at no charge. Some of the older female marksman athletes from the new former Russian countries came every day. It was a revolving door with 14 hour days with up to a 3 hour wait for athletes to have their hair cut. There were four teams of cosmetologist professionals, all ethnicities, from a multitude of salons and barber shops from across metro-Atlanta. Because of the security, especially after the bombing in Olympic Park, stylists were not able to bring shears in and out of the Olympic village area. Shears dulled quickly when rotated through different stylists cutting the thick healthy hair of athletes of all ethnicities. There were many problems with the shears, clippers and trimmers as they were shared among the different cutters.

The Design Essentials company of Atlanta kept everything running smoothly considering the fast pace and language barriers. Bonnie kept all the tools working like each individual stylist or barber wanted their tool to work. She learned a lot about customizing, innovating and some DIY tricks using what tools and supplies that were on hand. The Olympics was the training ground for the on the job ingenuity that has become the hallmark of Bonnie's career.

Group photo of some of the participants in the 2019 Sharpeners Jam in Atlanta, GA. This was the 21st Sharpeners Jam.

To foster this outside the box thinking in other sharpeners Bonnie began the Sharpeners Jam two years later in 1998. It began with three sharpeners sharing ideas. It has grown to be the oldest and largest sharpening conventions of its kind in the world. Sharpeners compete to see who can share the best ideas used in their sharpening businesses. Many of the hacks and ideas in this book came from this group of sharpeners. Some of the ideas are credited to them. Other ideas were presented so long ago and have been used so many years that she was unable to attribute the hack to the original sharpener. If one of your ideas is copied here, the author apologies to those who have contributed to her knowledge. Most likely more than one person has improvised in the same way. As Solomon said, *"There is nothing new under the sun."* (Ecclesiastes 1:9b NIV) It is true. All knowledge is built on someone else's idea.

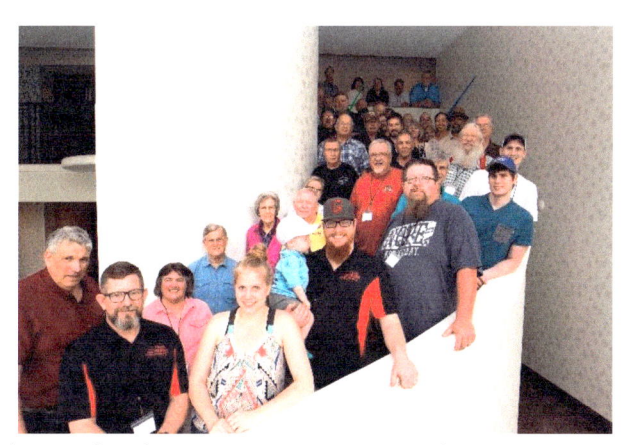

Bonnie continues to sharpen, train and learn. She is considered by many to be one of America's leading experts in the field of shear sharpening. This was evidenced when she became the first woman to receive the top score in an international shear sharpening certification. Her sharpening knowledge has been enhanced by classes with shear factory sharpeners from four countries. She is now in the process of furthering her knowledge with a trip to Solingen, Germany where shear manufacturing originated.

Bonnie has already begun work on her second book on shears. In addition in cooperation with a Spanish sharpener she will co-author a Spanish translation of this book. Please look for upcoming works from this author.

Made in the USA
Columbia, SC
29 April 2025